CONTENTS

Preface

Embedded in the deepest recesses of the human heart is the desire to look and feel our best. The quest for a flat, toned abdomen is one of the most sought after possessions of modern women. Woven into our emotional wellbeing is the desire to look and feel our best, sadly most lack the knowledge to obtain this priceless gift.

A new ground breaking and scientifically proven weight loss eating plan has been discovered which specifically targets stomach fat. Stomach fat can be incredibly resilient; visceral fat (stomach fat) is the most dangerous form of fat due to its proximity to vital internal organs and its toxic composition. It is indicative of increased risk of heart disease, strokes, type 2 diabetes and other metabolic conditions. Fortunately scientific research has recently identified the key components necessary to remove this unsightly bulge.

The central premise of "How to get a flat stomach in 30 days" is that reverting back to nature with a combination of pure, organic foods and eliminating all of the processed stuff is the key to your success. Shifting the body's chemistry from a toxic (acidic) state to a more natural (alkaline) state will create profound changes both physiologically and physically.

Now, for the first time, all the winning pieces of the formula come together. Devised by experts and combined with over 20 years of meticulous research and experience, I have distilled this knowledge into an easy to follow, step by step, day by day plan which will not only lead you towards a flat stomach but to a more healthy, happy and energised you. I also address and correct the thorny issue of emotional eating, offering easy to follow guidelines on how to correct it once and for all.

The techniques shown in "How to get a flat stomach in 30 days" have proven to be virtually 100% successful for those who genuinely apply its principles. Discover the fascinating facts about the foods you eat. The good news is that this book gives you all of the tools to obtain a flat stomach in 30 days and keep it!

This revolutionary weight loss plan offers:
- The 4 Golden rules to permanent weight loss which will give you that slender toned body you have dreamed of.
- The definite weight loss eating plan.
- The 8 super foods which will have you looking and feeling great.
- "Mind games" - precise strategies to help you mentally adapt to changing your lifestyle forever.
- A comprehensive "21 day Bikini blitz"

This book promises you "your best ever shape" and you will not be disappointed, because it really works!

Kevin Sheridan, August 2011

Disclaimer

The author and the publisher are not liable or responsible to any person or entity for any damage caused or alleged to be caused directly or indirectly by the information contained in this book.

Kevin is a personal trainer. He presents this book to you based on 20 years of his research and experience. Before you embark on this challenge you must consult your doctor/physician and get clearance from him/her as to precisely what you are permitted to do. The author insists you are monitored by your doctor and a qualified personal trainer throughout the programme. Partaking in this programme is done entirely at your own risk.

About the Author

Kevin Sheridan is an NCEF qualified personal trainer with over twenty years of experience specializing in weight loss, toning and fitness. He lives and works in Dublin where he is a full time personal trainer. He has written articles for Woman's Way magazine and is a frequent contributor to Spirit radio (50,000 listeners) where he speaks on weight loss. Kevin has featured on the "Four Live" programme on the Irish television station RTE1 as a weight loss expert. He is also a part time college lecturer specialising on fitness and healthy lifestyles and is currently involved in drawing up a syllabus on health and fitness for Irish schools.

STEP 1

THE PRINCIPLES

1

Introduction

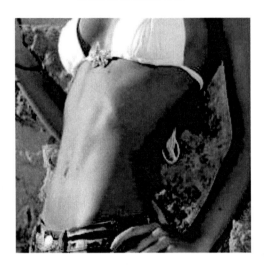

Who Am I and Why Should You Listen to Me?

I am sure you are thinking "another book about weight loss and achieving a flat stomach" and why should you listen to me? I am a qualified personal trainer and for most of my adult life have been helping people like you to successfully lose weight. For over two decades I have been involved in the weight loss and fitness industry as an expert who can deliver results. I have set up a highly successful personal training business specializing in weight loss, written two books, appeared on radio and TV, and I am the founder of a weight loss clinic, giving seminars on the truth about weight loss. My clients range from elite athletes to celebrities to people from all walks of life wishing to lose that frustrating stomach. Let me share my story.

"The dream was to have a flat stomach….."

Many years ago my life was a mess. I was 14 Kg (30 pounds) overweight, my school reports were appalling and my relationships with my family were very poor. In short; I was miserable. It is only when you experience firsthand the pain of being overweight that you can truly understand what overweight people are going through. The self-loathing, the insecurities, the "poor me" syndrome, the constant camouflaging of the ever expanding waistline, hiding behind masks of "I don't care" if someone makes an unflattering remark about your size while secretly it is a sword piercing through your heart.

"Little did I know that my dream was about to come true..."

Little did I realise that out of this despair was to come my true vocation in life, finding a permanent solution to weight loss. I searched in vain for years trying to discover how to lose this paunch. I tried everything on the market but to no avail. I had been given glimpses of the answer, so I embarked on a search that would cross continents, bringing me to moments of despair, hope and a new beginning. I began by tracing back through history, studying what the greatest teachers handed down. I have read hundreds of books, attended seminars, taken courses and scoured the internet in a search to uncover the universal principles for creating a flat stomach. These principles and techniques have not only worked for me but they have helped hundreds of people to achieve their ideal shape. All of these results are also possible for you. I know for a fact that you too, can make incredible changes to your shape, stomach and wellbeing.

The fact is that anyone can produce these kinds of results once you decide to believe the techniques work and begin to put into practice the principles shown in this book. By applying the principles and strategies, assimilating them into your lifestyle, and using them every day you too can literally transform yourself beyond your wildest dreams.

"...bit by bit, all the pieces began to fall into place..."

My vision was to share this information with you, aware of the pain and suffering that you may have endured by offering a simple to understand, step by step solution and helping you to customize each pillar of the weight loss formula. It is my sincerest hope that this book will enable you to pursue your dreams of achieving a flat stomach and bring joy and happiness into your life.

We all are governed by the same laws, these natural laws are the bed rock of the universe, they are so exacting that we have no difficulty in achieving incredible feats in our lives, yet our weight remains is out of control. The battle to achieve a flat stomach is primarily won or lost in your mind. Gaining mastery over your mind is one of the most crucial steps you can take in the battle to lose weight.

What have my clients have said about my method?

"It has changed my life and I will never look back ever" (Primary School Teacher)

"It been a great experience" (Special needs Teacher)

"Lighter, happier, being noticed and good company now" (Retired accountant)

"Life with fruit is fantastic" (Professional Chef)

"I've never felt so good; my confidence has gone through the roof" (Businessman)

"Lose weight, you bet!" (Tour Bus Driver)

"Do the right thing and the right thing happens" (Secondary School Teacher)

"Overall excellent, very beneficial and really helped me and my family" (Businesswoman)

"Very enjoyable" (Primary School Teacher)

"Hard work does not kill you, but it really pays off" (Driving Instructor)

"I would recommend it to my friends and family, very professional" (Housewife)

"Much easier than I expected, I feel great afterwards - both mentally and physically" (Housewife)

Towards a Flatter Stomach

Modern day society has become obsessed with its quest for body perfection. This book contains a unique synergy of ideas, methods and techniques which are put together in an easy to follow format. The individual components of this system are based on the formula MERC.

To use a simple analogy, trying to obtain a flat stomach in 30 days is like a chair with four legs; remove one leg and what happens? You need all four legs!! The MERC formula is what makes this book unlike any other diet book you have ever read.

This formula is the central premise of the book. By the same token, there is a proper combination of nutrition and exercise which must be tailored to your specific requirements.

I know these principals work for two reasons; firstly, I have tested and proved them on myself. Secondly, I have taught this system for the last 15 years and it has worked for every single person who has seriously applied these principles to their lives. One of the most important discoveries I made is that knowledge is the key. We live in a technological age where knowledge is at our fingertips, yet with so much conflicting theories being offered it can be confusing. By reverting back to our primal tendencies, we can identify the natural order in which we function. By respecting and meeting these requirements as nature intended a profound wisdom on weight loss is gained. As medicine and nutrition advances in an attempt to supply an "instant" cure, these findings generally take us away from what nature intended. As we become more exposed to toxins in our daily lives, we need to revert back to the tried and tested formulas which take into account the many other human facets which must be factored in to the overall equation. Take for example digestion, which is an integral part of achieving a flat stomach. If the digestive system is impaired it will lead to a multitude of problems. Once proper food combinations are adhered to, it allows for the easy absorption and release of the nutrients and for minerals to be dispersed properly. Foods which have been chemically altered, may be difficult to digest, hence they become trapped causing that bloated feeling, a toxic build up and inevitably weight gain.

Extensive research carried out by the Swedish scientist Are Waerland pinpointed that the body's ability to digest food lies in the efficiency of its three daily cycles.
1. The Appropriation cycle (noon to 8pm) Eating & digesting
2. The Assimilation cycle(8pm to 4am) Extracting nutrients
3. The Elimination cycle(4am to noon) Getting rid of waste

Protein has many powerful benefits for weight loss. Once you rebalance your carbohydrate intake and replace some of the carbohydrates with protein, your body will become a fat burning furnace. This was clearly shown in a 1999 study conducted at the Research Department of Human Nutrition in Copenhagen, Denmark. In this study, overweight and obese volunteers were put on either a high-carbohydrate diet (protein consisted of 12 per cent of their total calorie intake) or a high protein diet (25 per cent of their daily calories were protein based). The study lasted for six months and its findings were surprising to many. The first group who consumed a diet rich in carbohydrates lost 11 pounds (4.9Kg) while the second group who consumed a high protein based diet lost up to 20 pounds (9 Kg). But here is the key: the group that consumed the high protein based foods lost 17 pounds (7.7Kg) of pure body fat, compared to the first group (those who on the high carbohydrate diet) who lost just 9 pounds (4Kg) of body fat.

Amazingly, the higher protein eating plan assists in removing the unsightly stomach bulge and has been found to be the most effective weight loss ally. What does this mean to you? Consuming a *correctly balanced* eating plan rich in protein can double your weight loss results!

Resistance training (weight training) is another important ally in the battle against stomach fat. A recent research study compared the effectiveness of two exercise and diet programs. Subjects taking part in the study were assigned to one of two groups.

- Group one followed a diet based on the traditional food pyramid (50-55% carbohydrate; 15-20% protein; less than 30% fat). They also did cardiovascular exercise 4-6 days per week at 50-75% of their maximal heart rate. Each workout lasted 30-60 minutes.
- Group two followed a diet that was higher in protein and lower in carbohydrate and fat. Their exercise program consisted of alternating resistance and cardiovascular interval training six days per week.

Body composition was assessed by dual x-ray absorptiometry (DEXA) scans before and after the 12-week training program. DEXA is an extremely accurate way to measure changes in body fat. It's far more reliable than the skin fold callipers or body fat scales often used in health clubs.

The results showed that subjects in group two (remember, these were the people who lifted weights, did more intense cardio, and ate more protein) lost more fat overall (-20.6%) than the normal group (-10.1%). They also gained 2 pounds of muscle (0.9 kilograms) while the cardio-only group, not surprisingly, lost muscle. More interesting still, abdominal fat dropped by 26% in group two, but by just 13.5% in group one. In other words, subjects in group two lost almost twice as much belly fat as those in group one. What does this mean for you? Resistance training <u>must</u> be included in any successful weight loss plan.

What is unique about this book?

As a personal trainer, one of the most surprising things about my job is listening to what the vast majority of my clients wanted: a flat stomach. This troublesome area is pivotal to acquiring a figure you can be proud off. It is the first place where excess fat resides and, once this extra padding becomes firmly lodged around your abdomen and oblique's, it somehow manages to make everything feel uncomfortable. Your clothes strain to the point of breaking free. This does very little for your self-esteem.

This book shows you the **fastest** natural weight loss plan which specifically targets stubborn stomach fat.

At the foundation of this system is a universal truth which governs us all: safe and permanent weight loss is directly related to releasing toxins and replacing these toxins with natural alternatives. The key to this system is that it works with your body in eliminating toxic residue. Your body automatically responds by shedding pounds - no more of that bloated feeling! This is a life style change not a temporary behavioural change.

I also introduce the MERC weight loss formula. Weight loss is a complex issue; general guidelines are misleading, each reader has their own unique physiological and physical make up, which they can use to adapt each piece of the weight loss formula.

This book gives you the most effective fat burning techniques available today. These programs can be specifically adapted to <u>your</u> goals and take into account <u>your</u> physiological and physical make up

Losing the extra weight is only part of the problem! Once you have lost it, it is important to keep it off. I will show you a flexible weight maintenance programme for retaining results. I also tackle the thorny issues of food composition and food time tables, which must be corrected for lasting success.

Once you have achieved your goals, this book will show you how to keep your achievements and maintain your great new look.

When you read this book, you will discover the real reason for gaining weight, why diets don't work and you will learn why your body immediately regains the weight you may have lost when dieting. Most importantly, you will learn how to correct the underlying reasons which have lead to your weight gain in the first place.

What you can expect:

Firstly, the eating plan is designed to energise you while simultaneously burning fat; secondly, the exercise routines will remove fat deposit sites leaving you with a flat stomach and a lean toned figure. As you adhere to the guidelines, you will notice how your whole body will be re-sculpted. The flat stomach eating plan and exercise routine will add muscle tonality.

If you apply the techniques in this book you can expect:
•   To achieve a flat stomach.
•   To lose up to 15 pounds of body fat.
•   To reshape your body.
•   To improve your energy.
•   To improve or regain your self-confidence.
•   To burn away fat deposit sites permanently.
•   To never be hungry.
•   To have a firm bottom.
•   To have slender thighs.
•   To improve your physical fitness.
•   To conquer emotional eating.
•   To improve your productivity.
•   To be happier.
•   To improve your well-being.

2

Fat Burning Chemistry

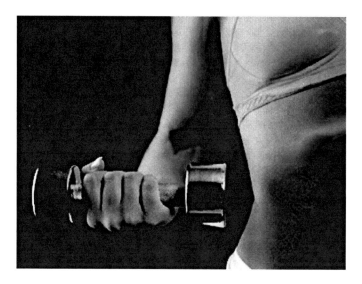

Introduction

Get ready to lose up to 15 pounds (6.8Kg) in 30 days! You are about to discover the greatest secret of all time relating to achieving a flat stomach and what really works. This book tackles all of the pieces of the jigsaw. A billion dollar industry has emerged offering you a quick fix with expensive drugs, surgery and pills. Do they really work? I have not found one in twenty years that has achieved lasting results. That is why I have turned to nature to provide the answers.

There is no one solution to achieving a flat stomach. Weight gain is a complex issue, finding a general solution resulting in one rule is fundamentally flawed. Yet there are precise laws which govern how you function. Understanding how your body works and responds is the key. Every reader has their own unique set of challenges, both mental and physical. The solution has been found, and it has been scientifically proven with virtually 100%

success for those who truly commit. You must prioritise this programme, approaching it with clarity and vision. You must concentrate on daily objectives and follow the exercise and nutritional instructions as outlined.

For most of the western world, modern eating fuelled by inactivity is contributing to producing nations where over 50% of the population are now overweight or obese. How can this happen even with all the advances of modern technology? The first task in my journey to find the answer was to uncover the latest medically proven research, test its validity and finally develop it into the most effective plan which specifically targets stomach fat.

The eating plan you are about to discover is a carefully designed nutritional package which is founded on the latest and most advanced science which encompasses a cleansing of the body's cells while simultaneously reducing your waistline. "How to Get a Flat Stomach in 30 Days" addresses and corrects the physical & physiological factors which have caused you to gain weight. As your body readjusts metabolically, it enables the burning of calories more efficiently. Having achieved your ideal stomach, you can choose from a variety of healthy foods to retain your results forever. In addition, you will discover the benefits of exercise; how to super-charge your metabolism while never having to worry about gaining weight. You will learn how to access that ever important physiological switch which has been handed down from the latest research which is designed to empower and motivate you to achieve what you once thought was impossible.

Weight Loss: the Facts

Some experts suggest the metabolism is the main reason for being overweight or emotional eating is the true cause of obesity. Some support the theory that excess weight is caused by genetics, while others recommend taking a new multi supplement or delving into deeply rooted physiological beliefs to unravel the truth. The truth is that weight gain is caused by a number of factors which may include some of the above. Understanding your physiological triggers, learning how you react to stress and what motivates are key ingredients for your success.

I knew that "How to Get a Flat Stomach in 30 days" was going to have to compete with numerous other books promising all sorts of wonderful concepts on how to lose weight. I knew that this book would have to have something unique that would allow it to stand alone, something which other books could not offer. At last, I have identified an eating plan which is grounded in the latest and most credible medical science and which offers the most realistic, satisfying eating plan that really works. The world's largest nutritional study confirmed the most effective method of weight loss is to eat lots of low-fat dairy products, lean meat, fish, beans and fewer foods which are starchy or high in refined sugar. White flour and rice should be removed from your eating plan.

The secret to keeping off those unwanted pounds is a **High Protein & Low GI** (Glycaemic Index) eating plan. The Glycaemic index of a food is a measure of its carbohydrate content and how easily it is converted to glucose. Foods with a low GI are slower to digest allowing you to feel full for longer. An international study of more than 900 adults and 800 children found that after 6 months, those on the high protein and low GI diet were 2 kg lighter than those on rival diets or high GI foods. The participants had already lost 11kg and were testing alternative approaches to maintain their ideal weight. Professor Arne Astrup of the University of Copenhagen, who led the study, found that the results suggested that official dietary advice was now redundant. His comments were surprising as he was one of the main enemies of the GI plan. "I expected in this trial it would make no difference, I am really surprised."

Vitamins & Minerals

Firstly, we will look at modern day eating. Research has found that modern day eating habits are generally unbalanced with an insufficient amount of critical minerals and vitamins. A balanced eating plan will include the following:

- Calcium (essential for bone growth & repair)
- Vitamin A (supports the immune system)
- Vitamin D (essential for bone growth and repair)
- Vitamin C (a powerful antioxidant which protects against heart and lung disease)
- Vitamin E (Reduces free radical activity)

- Folic Acid (protects against heart disease and nerve damage)
- Iron (is required by the body to form haemoglobin, the compound within the red blood cells that transports oxygen)
- Magnesium (Crucial for muscle contraction)

Vitamins may be sourced in small amounts. They play a key role in the metabolising process. Your daily vitamin requirements which are found in the flat stomach eating plan are as follows:

- Biotin: found in Oatmeal, milk and beans.
- Vitamin A: found in Carrots, milk, dairy products, potatoes.
- Vitamin B6: found in Meat, poultry, fish, nuts.
- Vitamin B12: found in Meats, eggs, liver, fish, cereal.
- Vitamin C: found in Citrus fruit, green vegetables.
- Vitamin D: found in fortified milk, egg yolks, salmon
- Vitamin E: found in Nuts, seeds, whole grains.

Minerals play an essential role in supporting healthy bones and teeth by creating a structural firmness. Nerve signals which are vital for brain and muscle functioning depend on calcium, magnesium, sodium and potassium. Zinc is crucial for body repair, renewal and development. The most important minerals and their sources are listed below:

- Calcium: dairy products, almonds, turnips
- Iodine: Seafood, seaweed
- Copper: Lobster, oysters, avocados
- Iron: Green leafy vegetables, whole grains, lean meat
- Magnesium: Spinach, rice, fruit
- Potassium: Orange juice, baked potato, bananas, nuts,
- Selenium: Grains, wheat germ, seafood, mushrooms
- Zinc: Seafood, wheat, dairy, beans

Weight Gain: How did this Happen to Me?

Here are the top 3 most likely answers.

1. Your Metabolism is underperforming: an eating plan consisting of convenience food or take away foods are the main reason for an underperforming metabolism.

2. Emotional eating: usually junk is the main culprit. This upsets your natural rhythms and cycles. It destabilises your blood sugars, creating spikes and dips. You literally become addicted to foods that have a large fat content, containing saturated fat, hydrogenated oils and empty calories. This type of food creates an imbalance of the neurotransmitters in the brain. Emotional eating is a conditional response to an emotional situation. We often associate pleasure or reward with certain types of food. Emotional eating hinges on a combination of two factors stress and upset which trigger a subconscious automated response to seek solace where possible.

3. Chemical addiction: once your taste buds have identified a certain taste, they will literally crave it. This leads us to one of the golden rules of weight loss: "what you eat you crave".

Flat Stomach Problem—Chemically Altered Foods

Nutritionists and health experts often talk about counting calories, some offer more insightful recommendations such as simple carbohydrates versus complex carbohydrates, but what does all of this mean to you? Most of these experts fail to mention the main culprit behind excess weight which is the chemically enhancing agents; these chemical additions create the addiction. This fast food industry is laden with manmade artificially enhancing agents known as flavour enhancers; they also contribute to a longer shelf life. Dairy and meat are often laden with growth enhancing hormones used to shorten the production time of beef and pork. Trans fat such as hydrogenated fats can be found in most manmade food and this type of artificial food will easily cause weight gain. The pasteurization of dairy products has become dependant on chemical agents. Digestive stress is a term used to describe the burdens of a toxic or acidic digestive system. An acidic digestive system will not break down food efficiently.

Foods which are infused with chemical components are man-made foods. These foods have pesticides, fertilizers and growth enhancing agents which when consumed lower your metabolic rate. There are over 10,000 chemicals which may be added to foods to increase their commercial value or to increase their shelf life, resulting in a dependency on this type of artificially flavoured food.

Making small changes to your daily eating plan can make a profound difference to your weight and wellbeing.

Break the cycle!

- Never allow yourself to get hungry! When your blood sugars drop, you feel ravenous, craving junk.
- By eating every two hours you will keep your blood sugars stable and avoid hunger.
- By weaning yourself off processed foods and switching to natural organic foods, your taste buds will readjust, in turn allowing your metabolism to function at its optimum level.
- Junk and processed foods clog up your metabolism, food particles become trapped in your intestine resulting in an underactive metabolic rate.
- The key to permanent weight loss is to reset your metabolism to function at its optimum level.

Diet supplements and meal replacements don't work long in the long term. Their claims of raising your metabolic rate, eliminating fluid, laxative Pills; thyroid enhancing supplements, growth hormones, creams, etc. should all be approached with caution. These mostly offer temporary solutions, not permanent results. Exercise is most beneficial, but it is only one part of the winning formula. Correct resistance exercises will target those problem areas, cardiovascular exercise adhering to the correct format will burn off those calories.

The most important factor in weight loss is establishing a correct eating plan. This will reset your metabolism, allowing it to burn calories effectively. Your blood sugars will stabilise. This is about changing your lifestyle, eating properly and finding an eating regime that you can live with for the rest of your life. The eating plan in this book will correct your eating patterns once and for all!

Flat Stomach Remedy

Excess insulin is one of the primary factors that make us overweight. The key to solving this is to control your insulin levels by eating low GI and high protein foods. For example: at breakfast if you take a bowl of oatmeal, add some non salted nuts or seeds. Alternatively you can have eggs on a slice of brown bread. For snacks you can have organic yogurt, avocado pear, a handful of non salted nuts. This way you are slowing down the rate at which the food is being broken down, preventing sudden rises and falls in your insulin level. By controlling your insulin level you help prevent fat being stored as an energy source. Low insulin foods (Low GI) include meat, fish, and dairy products. The secret is to maintain a stable blood sugar level throughout the day.

Balancing blood sugars will prevent you from craving carbohydrates and junk food. If you feel tired or hungry it may suggest that your blood sugar has dipped. Eating every two hours will ensure that this does not happen. If you feel hungry or bloated after a meal it may indicate that your body has produced too much insulin and the food combining was incorrect. Abundance of insulin helps to make you fat.

Eating protein often throughout the day will stabilise your blood sugars and allow you to feel full. When you skip meals, your body goes into panic mode and stores everything you eat as fat to conserve energy supplies. Eating protein little and often will prevent the craving for junk.

Water is Key for a Flatter Stomach!!

Drinking 2 litres of water a day will not only improve your digestive system but also support weight loss. Your kidneys require water to work effectively and to remove waste from your body. If there is a water shortage, your kidneys seek help from your liver. The main function of the liver is to use stored fat as an energy source. This diminishes your livers primary function which impairs its fat-burning potential. Another fat-burning technique is to change from drinking normal tea to herbal tea or green tea. Green tea has been found to stimulate the metabolism resulting in more calories being burned.

Food stays in your stomach for up to 4 hours until the end mixture is released into the small intestine. Low alkaline foods pass quickly through the digestive process, but red meat, which is more acidic, takes longer to digest producing high levels of acidity. Low alkaline foods (natural foods) place very little stress on the digestive process. It is important to note that your stomach reacts to emotions: when you feel stressed, more acid is produced effecting your natural digestion.

The biggest obstacle to weight loss is keeping the weight off permanently. Resetting your metabolism is one of the most crucial stages of this programme. No other weight loss programme addresses this problem as thoroughly as this programme does.

One difficulty with many of the weight loss books released lately is they are written by authors who were never overweight themselves. How can they relate to the challenges that you and I are faced with? It is simple to write down theories; it is completely different when you are the one going through the nightmare of being overweight with a protruding paunch. They did not experience the effects of excess weight on your self esteem, of feeling different, of trying to camouflage your weight by hiding under layers of clothing.

When you severely restrict your food intake, your body retains these fat deposits sites as a survival mechanism, only releasing them after months of starvation. With this programme, you will not lose structural fat or muscle. The resistance exercises will tone up those problematic areas while ensuring a flat stomach is complemented by a slender yet defined look. When you have achieved your ideal flat stomach, you will move onto the maintenance programme, burning excess calories. You will have broken the chains of emotional eating which have sabotaged your hopes and dreams and finally lay to rest fast and convenient food paradox. You will look and feel better than you ever have in your entire life – this is my promise to you.

How are we Going to Do It?

Much has been written of the merits of exercise, but exercise is only one part of the equation, so the main focus of this book is twofold.

The first step is concerned with getting clean. We must eliminate all toxins form your eating plan. This is the foundation stone on which the whole process is based on. You will never achieve a flat stomach on a toxic eating plan. Your body stores toxins in your fat cells; you must first remove these toxins. With an insufficient daily calorie count (i.e. starving yourself) you will feel miserable and lethargic! You body reacts by going into starvation mode which immobilises the fat. While some diets permit unlimited amounts of particular foods it creates an imbalance of insufficient critical minerals and vitamins which regulate dynamic cellular equilibrium. Toxicity will ensure you feel miserable, soft and pudgy.

The second step is to transform yourself by addressing the physiological work you will need to do to achieve a flat stomach. This work will dismantle any mental and emotional barriers which must be removed for lasting change. Crucially, you need to understand the importance of and the methodology of changing the self-limiting beliefs, controlling fears and negative habits which were holding you back. Finally you will be given the latest in cutting edge technology regarding nutrition and exercise which will ensure your success. It is like the numbers in a combination lock, you need them in the right order & sequence to unlock your formula.

If you apply all of the principles and techniques covered in this book you will achieve a flat stomach. It is natural to encounter obstacles along the way, remember these are only temporary. Let's begin with uncovering the truth about achieving a flat stomach!

3

Stomach Fat - The Secret Revealed

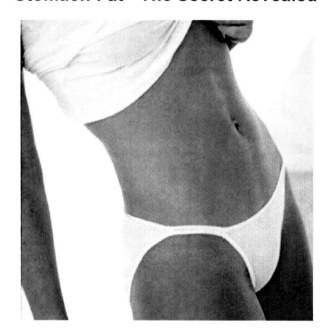

The Fat Factor – The Basics

Dietary fat is an essential component of a balanced eating plan. It assists in regulating your metabolism; it supports the structure of the cell membranes, it also provides insulation and improves the efficiency of your immune system. If we examine some of the healthiest eating plans in the world today, we find evidence that fat is an integral component of their daily eating plan. Many of us have been programmed to believe that all fats are undesirable. Not so!

It is a startling fact that since Americans embraced the "low-fat" mentality, obesity levels have steadily increased to epidemic levels. It is estimated that over 65% of Americans and 50% of the UK population are currently considered overweight or obese. Medical scientists rushed to probe these alarming statistics. How

18

could this be? Finally, it was discovered that people misunderstood the nutritional requirements of a balanced eating plan and had substituted carbohydrates for fat. This was the catalyst responsible for the low carbohydrate craze which swept through America. Carbohydrates where being blamed for our ever expanding waistlines, this combined with a more sedentary lifestyle fuelled the weight loss frenzy. It has been scientifically proven that high-carbohydrate diets contribute to the formation of body fat while certain types of natural "fats" assist in weight loss.

Fifty years ago, obesity was unheard of. What has happened in the intervening years? Society back then was self sufficient. They planted vegetables, harvested their own crops, and dairy produce was natural (without any modern chemicals). Animals roamed free eating unfertilised grass. Growth hormones, pesticides and fertilizers were not invented. As society became more "instant", manufactures catered for their needs by reducing the natural life cycle of meat and vegetables, thus offering customers an instant response. By injecting meat and poultry with growth hormones, antibiotics and a combination of artificially enhancing chemicals, this enabled the produce to be ready in a shorter time frame. Modifications were made to the pasteurization of dairy products, removing essential enzymes and minerals so these dairy products would have a longer shelf life.

All about Fats

Fats can be generally broken into two categories: "good" fats and "bad" fats.

Good Fats

Good fats are at the very core of "How to Get a Flat Stomach in 30 Days", they are the unsaturated variety: polyunsaturated oils and monounsaturated oils and fat which are necessary for your overall emotional and physical wellbeing. They support maximizing weight loss and should be stored correctly as they may spoil due to their natural chemical sensitivity.

Good fats assist in energy production and play a critical role in regulating your immune system. These desirable fats may be sourced from: Unsalted nuts, wild fish, egg yokes, avocados, tuna, salmon and flaxseeds. Good fats assist in mineral and vitamin distribution, thus supporting a cleaning role for the blood cells. These fats cannot be manufactured by your body so they must be sourced elsewhere. Once consumed, they are immediately used in the maintenance of healthy cell membranes and they assist in the development of long lean muscle.

Did you know?
Good fats also improve the texture of your skin and hair.

Omega 9 (found in olive oil, non salted nuts and avocados) is most favourable. Desirable fats act as an appetite suppresser which also help fight against heart disease, arthritis. Recent studies have forged a direct link between fish oil as a remedy to an array of stomach problems. They stimulate the release of cholecystokinin which is a hormone located in the stomach which signals to the brain not to eat more as it is full. Good fats regulate the balance of insulin and glucagon. When foods high in sugar are consumed, insulin is released to remove excess sugar from your body. If sugary foods are constantly consumed, it will result in excess insulin being present resulting in levels of Glucagon (the hormone required to burn body fat) being impaired.

Bad Fats

Bad fats prevent your metabolism from functioning correctly, while assisting in the build up of fatty acids around artery walls resulting in high blood pressure, heart attack and stoke. Bad fats fall into two categories.

1.   Saturated fats found in animal products such as salami sausages, cream, butter and full fat cheeses.

2.   Trans fats (also know as hydrogenated fats) this type of fat is manmade and has no nutritional benefits. Hydrogenated fats are chemically altered to remove the desirable fat content from its structure and replace it with undesirable fat. These fats were invented in the early 1900's and were first used to make margarine. This type of fat should be

completely eliminated from your eating plan. Hydrogenated fats can be found in most artificial cooking oils (if in doubt use pure olive oil which is always natural). Hydrogenated fats can be found in crisps, corn bread, biscuits, cakes, chocolate bars, cereals and crackers.

Fats can be identified in general as desirable or undesirable by their form at room temperature. Desirable fats are generally soft at room temperature as undesirable fats such as butter or margarine are solid at room temperature.

You can extend this theory to food on the shelves of your supermarket. If you baked a muffin at home how long do you think it would last before it spoiled? Probably a few days! How is it then that a muffin on a supermarket shelf can have a "best before" date of several weeks into the future? The only way this can be the case is if hydrogenated fats are used in the manufacture of the muffin. Hydrogenated fats are generally used to make processed food more "solid" and extend their shelf life.

Stomach Fat – The Facts

The primary reason you are carrying excess weight is caused primarily by what you eat, when you eat and your lifestyle rather than any mitigating circumstances. Often blame is directed towards genetics or a multitude of other excuses but this is rarely the case. When your body fat percentage stabilises for a period of one or more years, you will develop adipose cells, capillaries, enzyme counts and hormone levels which support your body fat percentage. Your body will monitor its fat reserves with a hormone called glycerol which signals your brain to go into defensive mode if there is a sudden drop in the level of your body fat.

Dieting Doesn't Work!

Dieting cannot work permanently; where else will you find people who starve themselves in an attempt to shed those unwanted pounds? It is common to feel miserable, irritable, depressed and lacking in energy. How long can a person cope with such discomfort? Many dieters are sabotaging their emotional and physical wellbeing for the sake of losing a few pounds of fluid, only to be regained when normal eating habits are returned to.

When you go on a diet, your system is thrown into turmoil, adding into the equation the "cold turkey" which dieters must endure as the chemical additives to which they have become addicted to are banned. This will almost guarantee failure but also it has a demoralising effect both mentally and physically. The constant searching for a permanent solution creates undue emotional pressure. What do you think about when you are dieting? The foods you love and miss. When you feel deprived, the source of this deprivation creates a longing for these forbidden foods!! How long can you hold out? A common trait with dieters is to binge followed by another resolution followed by another break out which fuels the self-loathing and disgust with yourself.

The 90/10 Rule

A much more sensible approach is to adopt the 90/10 rule which states that 90% of the time you adhere to the given format and 10% of the times you are allowed indulge. A gradual shift is far more sustainable. One to two pounds per week is the recommended level. Your body will respond by remodelling its adipose cells and capillaries to match. It is crucial to lose body fat and not metabolically active muscle. How can this be achieved? By incorporating light weight training into your activities two or three per week. Eliminating saturated fats from your daily eating plan and limiting your carbohydrate intake will prove most beneficial. Do you want a quick-fix or long lasting results?

Three Kinds of Body Fat

Structural Fat

Structural fat is found around organ parts, its role is to protect the organs and arties. It acts as a cushion for the joints. Structural fat is necessary for your health and wellbeing. With some weight loss programs, it is this type of fat which is removed first, often leaving a person looking gaunt. Surprisingly, when a person goes on a diet they lose structural fat, subcutaneous fat and lean muscle. It may also accelerate the aging process as the skin loses its elasticity, leaving the person on the diet looking gaunt, pale and miserable. The problem areas that were hoped would be targeted remain unchanged.

22

Subcutaneous Fat

Subcutaneous fat is found just under the skin and is used as a fat reserve. It is mostly found in various "pockets" around the body. In women it is located around the mid section, thighs and triceps. Normal fat reserves are an energy source. This type of fat is stored as an emergency mechanism, activated only by the threat of starvation. A moderate amount of subcutaneous fat is desirable (12% - 15%) as it supports the proper functioning of your immune system, but excess amounts can cause disfiguration of the body shape and may lead to lower back problems.

Visceral Fat

Visceral fat is the fat we are primarily targeting. It is found mostly deep within in the stomach region. Visceral fat is the most dangerous type of body fat as this is where toxic residues hide. Due to its high levels of toxicity when it is released it goes directly into the blood stream or the liver and has been directly linked to diabetes, heart attack, high blood pressure, strokes and some forms of cancer. The higher the levels of visceral fat found in your body, the higher the risk of contacting one of the above ailments.

Visceral fat is easy to put on but also easy to remove. Recent finding have found a direct link between weight loss and the reduction of visceral fat. Visceral fat is easier to lose than subcutaneous fat and the latest research suggests that the ideal approach to remove visceral fat is to increase your physical activity and decrease your intake of sugar and refined carbohydrates, substituting complex carbohydrates and protein (such as lean meats) in place of the heavy starchy carbohydrates. Limit your intake of alcohol to 4 units per week and try consuming polyunsaturated and monounsaturated fats in place of hydrogenated fats and Tran's fats.

How can we remove Visceral Fat?

The central premise of this book revolves around protein as the scientifically proven food source which keeps you full between meals. Cardiovascular activity supported by an eating plan rich in protein and desirable fats will remove several pounds of visceral fat over a period of months. The recommended weekly activity is between 30 to 40 minutes of nonstop exercise four to five times per week.

A common misconception is to believe that dieting alone will remove this unwanted fat tissue, it won't, and it must be removed by cardiovascular exercise. Remember: fat is essentially stored energy and it must be burned off! People who live a sedentary existence are prone to alarming levels of visceral fat. It will decrease your resistance to insulin which in turn may cause type 2 Diabetes. If you start to lose visceral fat your body eliminates toxins which are held within the visceral fat tissue thus enabling you to control high blood pressure and minimises the risk of cardiac problems or strokes. The more visceral fat you lose, the flatter your stomach becomes.

The two crucial components necessary to remove visceral fat are:
1. A well balanced eating plan, rich in desirable fats
2. Exercise: both aerobic & anaerobic activity.

The key is keep your cell membrane healthy, desirable fats are building blocks for providing more oxygen to the cells, ensuring that they do not age faster or are susceptible to the ravages of disease. The single worst thing you can do is to consume undesirable fats, when consumed they turn to a hard sticky substance which becomes clogged in the cell membrane.

Junk and convenience food are laden with artificial flavouring, colouring, toxic substances, and preservatives while hydrogenated fats and trans fats are always lurking just under the surface. Once your taste buds require a taste for this type of food they become addicted to the chemical composition therefore requiring more of it. This is where the addiction begins. This is the surest way to malnourish yourself while piling on extra pounds; it can also lead to a number of physiological and physical factors like depression and the erosion of your self-confidence. This type of food can cause degenerative diseases, impede the efficiency of the reproduction of your brain cells; and reduce the strength of your immune system. It can also result in cancer causing agents being dispersed throughout your body due to the chemical residue left by this type of food. Don't even think of going down the "Fat Free" or "Lite" road. It is only short for "Chemical avalanche".

Soda Craze!

Fizzy drinks are another name for glucose in its purist form. Glucose is pure energy that gets converted straight into fat unless it is used immediately. Don't get sucked into the "low calorie" or "diet" notion of fizzy drinks, it is a marketing ploy, and it's just sugar and chemicals you are consuming. Choose natural water instead. Trans fat leaves a residue of toxicity in the fatty tissue of your body. This food is designed to make you FAT. The worst offenders are the fast food companies. This type of food is rubbish, not only is it empty calories, it also may affect your serotonin levels (which effect your happiness) leaving you bloated, full of chemical reactions and miserable. What if I can show you a way to solve this? Read on!!

There are many contributing factors why YOU gained weight, both physiologically and physically. The central message in this book is to find YOUR solution. This is the first step which must be taken to establish weight loss, regardless of all of the other ingredients.

Saber-Tooth Tiger and You

Millions of years ago, our ancestors survival depended on their ability to respond immediately to impending danger. In order to escape from the jaws of a ravenous saber-tooth tiger, they relied on a defence mechanism which overrides all rational thinking. The famous "fight or flight "syndrome was founded. Today, you are equipped with the same neurological response. You may not have to face off a ravenous beast but you may have to deal with a demanding boss, partner or life situation. When experts refer to stress, they differentiate between the two different types: Acute or Chronic. The temporary stressful situation has no major long term implications; on the contrary it can have a positive effect allowing a more assertive response. However when a temporary stressful situation becomes long term (chronic) is when cracks begin to appear. Your body cannot distinguish the difference between stress and a life threatening situation, when your brain feels your life is under threat; it triggers an immediate response from your central nervous system. The central nervous system is broken down into voluntary and involuntary actions. The voluntary responses are controlled by your conscious mind; while involuntary actions work independently of your rational mind to which you have no control over.

What does this have to do with a flat stomach?

If this threat passes, your central nervous system signals a return to normal functioning. The involuntary nervous system regulates your bodies breathing, digestion and blood circulation. They return to their normal functioning only when the threat has passed and without your input. Here's what happens:

The Chemistry of Acute Stress

Stress responses start in your central nervous system. Your central nervous system is broken down into two distinct categories: Voluntary and Involuntary.

Your central nervous system responds to signals which are received from your conscious mind (voluntary). While your involuntary nervous response functions independently. For example if you wish to walk across the road, your voluntary nervous system will put in place the actions which are necessary to complete the task. This will cause no obstruction to your normal bodily functioning, you will continue to breathe, digest etc. These normal bodily functions are working automatically without any input of you consciously having to remind yourself to breathe. Within the involuntary nervous system there are two distinct systems working: the nervous system sympathetic (SNS) and the parasympathetic nervous system (PNS). The sympathetic nerves mobilize energy for the 'Fight or Flight' reaction during stress, causing increased blood pressure, breathing rate, and increases blood flow to muscles in response the imminent danger which is presented, and the second (PNS) responds by having a calming influence on the situation. For example if you are crossing the road and notice a car rapidly approaching, your heart responds by pumping blood faster though your veins, your begin to hyperventilate as you rush to safety, your brain has identified an immediate threat to your life and engages your involuntary nervous system.

- Once a stressful situation has been identified, a substance called corticotrophin releases adrenaline and cortisol into your system.
- Cortisol increases the levels of fat and glucose in your blood stream.
- Your blood flow from the heart increases, resulting in a rise in blood pressure as your arties narrow.
- The digestion system shuts down; in response to the liver releasing glucose.
- Muscles become tense as breathing becomes faster.
- Your pupils dilate as you focus on the impending danger.
- You become more alert.
- Adrenaline is released which increases your heart beat by respond by beating at twice its normal rate

These responses happen instantaneously to get you out of danger. Once the danger has passed, (acute or short term) your (PNS) reacts by releasing calming hormones which enable your body to return to its normal rhymes.

The Chronic Symptoms of Long Term Stress

The major difference between acute stress and chronic stress is that acute stress has a short lifespan. Once you become engaged in a long term difficult situation, it paves the way for chronic stress to set in. It is important to understand that your body cannot differentiate between acute or chronic stress; it reacts the same way so when the situation becomes prolonged there is no calming period. Your central nervous system keeps responding as it's programmed to by keeping you in a heightened state of anxiety. Once your bodies stress mechanism has been activated and is kept in this state of heightened sensitivity, the harder it becomes for you to switch off. This is where it becomes physically and mentally dangerous. Stress is becoming one of the major factors that can trigger an array of medical conditions. Here's how it works.

In stressful situations, the adrenal gland releases an abundance of Cortisol. Usually, cortisol's primary role is to regulate the blood pressure and cardiovascular activities while insuring the metabolism is working properly. The occasional release of cortisol can be absorbed without any negative side effects. If cortisol levels remain high, your body adapts to this level of stress.

Here is the killer: This is what contributes to the fat around the middle: High cortisol levels creates craving and increases your appetite so good supplies of fuel are ready when needed. Cortisol and adrenaline are the two main stress hormones. When insulin production is increased, it overrides a response from the adrenalin hormone to burn fat resulting in signalling to your body to store fat in its anticipation of future emergences. Excess cortisol weakens the immune system and increases your heart rate in anticipation of the looming disaster. An oversupply of cortisol can destabilise your neurotransmitters which control your serotonin levels (happy hormones) making you prone to depression. When a stressful situation becomes chronic you enter the resistance stage. The symptoms are:

- Lack of interest in life.
- Feeling overwhelmed.
- Lack of interest in sex.
- Headaches.
- Bad moods continuously.
- Feeling of despair.
- Lack of appetite.
- Disrupted sleeping patterns.
- Exhaustion.
- Difficulties with concentration.

Cortisol and Your Stomach

It is common to spend years in the resistance stage. The main difficulty is that when cortisol is constantly present, your fat cells (in particular in the stomach region) are receptive to cortisol which allows them to increase in size. Studies have found Cortisol increases your appetite, specifically for high sugar content foods. Remember the last time you felt really stressed? What did you go for? I'm betting it was junk food!

Cortisol requires your body to store fat as an energy reserve around the stomach region.

28

This is nature's way of providing energy for the next impending emergency.

Stress Busting Calmers: 5 Secret Techniques.

The key factor in terms of weight control is to think about how your body reacts to stress and try to rebalance your life. Factoring in a time management structure where you allocate time each day to removing stressful situations as much as possible.

Secret 1: The Coffee myth

Caffeine may cause important enzyme systems to malfunction; caffeine can lead to poor concentration, dehydration, kidney problems, poor skin and may lead to cancer causing agents been released into your system. It may also desensitise certain nerve receptor sites. Caffeine is acidic (Toxic) which may result in your body producing fat cells in order to protect your organs from this. Coffee is artificially enhanced; it is full of pesticides.

Secret 2: Sleeping beauty

Sleep deprivation reduces the size of your brain cells. It is one of the most effective torture routines ever devised. In a sleep deprived state your moods reflect how you feel!! Scientists suggest that in order to function at your optimum level, you need 7 to 8 hours a night. In recent times, sleeping patterns have decreased with most people getting between 6 and 7 hours due to the internet and other stimuli. The paradox is that we both need sleep and resist it. Mostly we struggle by on less sleep in the hope of refuelling our sleep gauge at the weekend. Sleep can slip down the ladder of our priorities as you juggle with the demands of modern living. When deprived of sleep, you are more likely to make flawed decisions and are prone to accidents. When in a sleep deprived state, it requires extra carbohydrates to sustain your energy levels. Recently, a study completed on the effects of stress found that if you increase your sleeping habits by 20 to 30 minutes daily, it will make a profound difference to your coping mechanisms. It has been found that a person who is experiencing sleep difficulties will require up to 30% more carbohydrates than someone who is not. Dr. Neal Kohatsu from the California department of health Services states "Even a modest increase in sleep duration has shown to have a clinically significant affect on weight". Sleep disorders may be caused by stress, nutritional difficulties, toxins and excess caffeine while other stimulants such as junk and processed foods can leave you nutritionally malnourished. Over the counter sleeping aids should be avoided as they will encourage continual usage. Remember the last time you felt exhausted? What did you crave?

Secret 3: Be wise and exercise

Studies have found that exercise will help reduce the feeling of anxiety and also remove the levels of cortisol in your bloodstream. Exercise has a unique way of changing the body's physiological and physical state. With the release of endorphins it will lift your mood regardless of how sombre it may be.

Secret 4: The key to misery is isolation!

When you feel challenged, the natural inclination is to lock yourself away worrying over the impending obstacle. By seeking out trustiest friends, they can provide clarity from an objective position.

Secret 5: Indulge - the pathway to happiness

Research has shown that people who engage in recreational activities regularly are more contented within themselves. Indulge in activities you enjoy be it a massage, a scented bath or any positive activity. Treat yourself!

The key is moderation, if you enjoy coffee allow one cup per day. One of the best ways to begin the day is with a cup of warm water with a squeeze of flesh lemon. It is a wonderful detoxifier, while cleansing the liver. It works wonders for your complexion and helps to combat free radical activity.

The foods which are on the flat stomach eating plan have been scientifically proven to be effective combination of carbohydrates, fats and proteins, providing you with a balanced and structured eating plan. It provides all the nutrients and vitamins required to stimulate your metabolism and increase your fat-burning potential. This eating plan also offers a caloric reduction which creates the calorie deficit. The food you consume will ensure more energy and noticeable improvements to your well-being while ensuring fat-loss.

Carbohydrates: The Truth

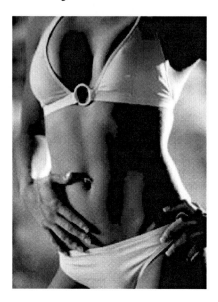

All about Carbs

Carbohydrates have the recipient of much bad publicity lately. What is there function? Many people want to know: Will I achieve a flat stomach if I cut carbohydrates?

The primary role of carbohydrates is as an energy source. When digested, they are transformed into glucose (sugar) which is released into your blood stream. Once there, it is used as energy source for the red blood cells and also supports the proper functioning of your central nervous system. If Glucose is not used up immediately, it is stored in the liver and muscles as glycogen which is another energy reserve. An eating plan rich in high fibre contents has been found to support fat reduction. One of the main benefits of an eating plan rich in fibre is that you feel full, which reduces the craving for junk food as it has a stabilising effect on your blood sugars.

Research has established a direct link between carbohydrates and the brain functioning at its optimum level, also your serotonin levels (the happy hormones) react positively to carbohydrates.

The aim of a balanced eating plan is to provide your body with all the nutrients necessary for its vital functions and systems to perform at their optimum levels. Each nutrient may be accessed through different foods, which is the primary reason for a balanced eating plan.

> **Did you know?** Protein, carbohydrates and fats are nutrients which have their own unique functions which enable you to operate at your correct level.

Without the necessary nutrients: carbohydrates, fats, protein, vitamins and minerals, your body immediately responds by underperforming. This is where conventional wisdom surpasses the latest diets. How much of our daily intake should be made up of carbohydrates? Research suggests that up to 40% of your daily food intake should consist of desirable carbohydrates. Do not be fooled by the marketing ploy of "low-carb" or "reduced-carb" products. Your body cannot absorb these refined carbohydrates with the same ease as it would natural foods. The most common mistakes are to believe that cereals, white breads, biscuits, white rice, bagels, muffins and pastries are supplying you with the essential minerals and vitamins you require.

> **Did you know?** Fruit is the most complete food source available; it is as close to the perfect food source by requiring minimal effort to digest.

Fruit is also high in enzymes and it passes through your digestive tract effortlessly, nourishing you with vital carbohydrates, fibre, minerals, fatty acids and also administering cancer fighting agents. Fruits main composition is water; so it assists your body in cleansing and detoxification.

Did you know? Fruit must be eaten on an empty stomach.

There are two main categories of carbohydrates and the key is to choose the right type.

Simple carbohydrates

Simple carbohydrates are made up of molecules of sugar. When consumed they immediately enter the blood stream, allowing for an immediate sugar rush. This instant rush may destabilise your blood sugars sending them soaring, but it is unsustainable and as your blood sugars tumble you will need to boost them again. Simple carbohydrates are found in sweets, cakes, fruit juices, processed foods, ice cream, carbonated drinks, and chocolate.

Complex carbohydrates

Complex carbohydrates consist of starch and fibre, which is the bedrock of a balanced eating plan. They have a different molecule structure, which enables them to be broken down slower, resulting in a lasting energy source which stabilises the blood sugars. Complex carbohydrates are not water soluble and require time to digest properly. Complex carbohydrates can be found in potatoes, brown rice and whole grains. These are desirable carbohydrates as they are packed with starch. Green vegetables such as spinach and broccoli are excellent sources of fibre.

Fibre is classified as essential ingredient in a balanced eating plan. It enables the transportation of digestible foods to pass through the intestine preventing bowl problems. Natural sources of fibre are fruit, vegetables and brown wholegrain bread.

The GI index

Simple carbohydrates have one or two molecules of sugar, while complex carbohydrates have a multiple number of sugar molecules. For greater clarification, a method known as the Glycaemic index was introduced in the 1980`s. This method ranked carbohydrates by the effect they have on blood sugars. Foods with a high index are rated with a glucose value of 100, the higher the number the faster it converts to glucose. Foods with an index reading of 70 and over are considered high GI, with foods between 50 and 70 considered medium and below 50 are considered low GI.

Foods which contain a High GI and a Low GI have the same intrinsic value for the food energy which we derive from them, both have a similar calorie count, but there is one major difference, foods with a high GI tend to be released quickly into your blood stream giving you a sudden boost of energy followed by a sudden low.

Carbohydrates with a low GI are gently released into your blood stream giving you a stable blood sugar level, allowing you a sustained energy level. Foods with a high GI tend to cause blood glucose levels to rise quickly and provoke a rapid insulin response. It also produces high levels of insulin, which in turn activates fat cell enzymes. These transport fat from your blood stream into fat cell storage which in turn creates more fat cells. When foods with a high GI are consumed, you will feel hungry shortly after.

Foods with a high GI, support your body in storing fat. Foods with a low GI will encourage your body to burn fat while sustaining your metabolism for longer periods.

High GI (undesirable for weight loss)	Low GI (desirable for weight loss)
• White bread	• Oatmeal
• Potatoes	• Fresh vegetables
• Processed vegetables	• Natural fruit
• Canned fruit	• Brown pasta
• Concentrated fruit juices	• Wild rice
• Fizzy drinks	• Organic eggs
• Biscuits	• Organic meat
• Savoury crackers	• Organic fish
• Popcorn	• Oats
• Crisps	• Dairy produce

Many years ago, the traditional eating plan was higher in natural starches and fibre. Latest research shows evidence that simple carbohydrates, most white flour, refined sugars and manmade foods with a high GI will cause the levels of glucose to rise and may provoke rapid insulin change. Carbohydrates with low GI, foods rich in natural origins, such as watermelon, fruit, wholemeal bread, wild rice and fresh vegetables cause a slower insulin response. By consuming complex carbohydrates, every two hours will allow your body to produce less insulin while avoiding the sugar Highs and Lows. Your food intake becomes better regulated.

The refining process tries to highlight the added benefits of certain undesirable foods by "added "or "extra" which is a marketing tool. These foods are mostly nutritionally barren. Remember the last time you consumed this type of food, how you felt?

A toxic eating plan can be recognised by bloating, excess weight, cellulite, dark circles under the eyes, poor skin texture, premature aging, nervous disposition, ulcers, poor concentration and feeling constantly lethargic.

Six Steps to an Instantly Slimmer You

Changing your eating habits need not be traumatic. Implementing small daily changes can have a profound impact on your health. The battle for losing weight is won or lost in your mind and by returning to natural food sources.

1. **Keep hydrated**. It is easy to fall into the trap of drinking fizzy drinks, tea and coffee. Try drinking two to two and a half litres of water daily. This has a flushing effect on toxins, literally flushing them out of your system. Alternatively drink herbal teas instead of tea and coffee. These are a wonderful source of antioxidants which help protect your body against the dangers of free radicals. You will feel terrific!

2. **Think about food.** Think about what you are going to eat, is it man made or is it natural? Eliminate habitual eating. I ask clients to keep a food diary, try writing down exactly what you eat for 3 days! It really focuses your mind. Avoid

processed foods if possible. Foods which are rich in vitamins and minerals nourish your body, enabling you to resist food craving. Alcohol is a sugar which promotes the production oestrogen in your blood stream, leading to the increase of fat storage cells around your stomach. It causes hydrochloric acid to rise in your stomach resulting in that bloating feeling. Alcohol will dehydrate you resulting in feeling lethargic and bloated.

3. **Limit carbohydrates.** We have become heavily reliant on heavy carbohydrates. Starch laden foods will diminish your energy levels. Try eliminating sugary cereals for breakfast, rolls for lunch and pasta or chips for dinner. By consuming so much starchy carbohydrates, you will feel lethargic, bloated and miserable. Carbohydrates are a wonderful source of energy when chosen wisely. Begin the day with oatmeal or fruit; add nuts or berries along with a herbal tea. Replace a pastry and coffee with a selection of fruit. Lunch; replace bread with lean protein rich foods like roast chicken salad or pesto with low fat cheese or salad sprinkled with roasted seeds or nuts. Finally in the evening have lean meat or wild fish, with a selection of green vegetables or wild brown rice.

4. **Fish.** Wild fish such as salmon or sea bass are great sources of omega-3 fatty acids. This has many positive effects on your heart, brain and joints while stabilising your blood sugars and maintaining your energy levels and moods.

5. **Five a day**. We have all heard that we must have five portions of fruit and vegetables a day. Blackberries, strawberries pears, apples, rhubarb and vegetables are packed full of vitamins. They have nourishing levels of nutrients such as vitamin c, selenium and fibre. There are many ways to ensure you get your five a day. Avoid microwaving; instead try steaming or a juicer. Use olive oil as a dressing to create a salad. Use Greek yogurt and pumpkin seeds as a snack before retiring to bed.

6. **Eliminate salt.** Too much salt will aggravate fluid retention, making you bloated and uncomfortable. There is a common misconception that salt will cause weight gain. The truth is

salt will cause water retention. By drinking 1 to 2 litres of water daily, you will excrete this water weight. Salt is an important source of sodium and iodine. Sodium assists with other minerals to support nerve stimulation and control water balance. It assists in carbohydrate usage. Consuming salt in its natural state will not cause a negative reaction but eating take away foods laden with salt may lead to high and potentially dangerous levels of sodium. Substituting herbs or natural dressings instead of salt will enhance flavours while maintaining your ideal sodium and iodine levels. If you must have salt, try the natural sea salt, this has the same module structure as table salt.

The Stomach Destroyer

Eliminating white sugar from your eating plan is at the very core of losing weight. This white poison infiltrates every modern type of food. Manufacturers know the benefits of concealing it in their products. Sugar in its natural state has many health benefits. The main issue with refined sugar is all the enzymes, vitamins and minerals have been removed through the refinement process. This refined sugar is added to foods to sweeten its taste and camouflage the nutritional content of what you are eating. Processed and convenient foods are laden with refined sugar and salt. Refined sugar is empty calories; it has no health benefits whatsoever. Excess sugar is stored in the liver, when this overflows it is released into the blood stream as fatty acids. These particles cling on to the walls of the arteries, over time it coagulates forming hardened arties restricting the blood flow through the arteries. In time this may lead to restricted blood flow resulting in cardiac arrest.

Did you know? Fruit is the ideal substitute for sugary snacks.

Each time sugar is consumed, with the exception of immediately after exercise, your blood sugar rises causing an insulin spike and your liver must balance the excess insulin by turning it into triglycerides (fat) which is deposited as fat reserves. The key to keeping your blood sugar level stable is to eat every two hours.

By eliminating simple sugar from your daily eating plan and substituting complex carbohydrates, it will have a stabilising effect on your blood sugars. Simple sugar also increases the size of your liver, and it can lead to numerous diseases and accelerates the aging process. As well as being highly addictive, refined sugar diminishes the role of valuable nutrients in the body. Remove refined sugar, processed fruit juices, pastries, and biscuits as well as the low fat foods. Don't be fooled by the common disguises of sucrose, maltose, lactose and fructose on food labels. These are all other names for sugar! It is also worth noting that the body tends to treat alcohol as a sugar when it metabolizes it, so you should treat alcohol as a sugar too.

Manufactures often re-label sugar with a multitude of names like syrup, fructose or corn syrup. Energy bars, cereals, cakes, yogurts, bagels, canned fruit are often laden with these types of undesirable sugar. The American journal of Clinical Nutrition conducted a study and found a direct link between eating refined sugar and obesity and diabetes.

The Truth about Achieving a Flat Stomach

If you have had difficulty in the past losing weight, the reason may lie in two nutritional components: <u>food composition</u> and <u>food time table</u>. "Composition" referrers to the ratio of carbohydrates, fats and proteins which are daily consumed and the "time table" involves the time at which you eat. Medical experts have only recently found the correlation between weight gain and food composition and time tabling. They have identified these two nutritional elements as being the bedrock of a successful weight loss plan.

Some experts suggest that by eliminating one particular food group (protein/carbohydrate or fat) it will accelerate your weight loss potential but at what cost? Your body has been designed to function with such precision that by omitting one food group can be detrimental to your wellbeing. Weight loss is achieved by carefully selecting the right type of foods which will ensure you get your necessary vitamins and minerals and eating at the correct time will speed up the fat burning process. By excluding certain food groups you will destabilise your blood sugars and hormonal balance. Vitamins and minerals help to regulate your metabolism. Seeing chiselled stomach muscles is entirely about reducing your body fat percentages.

All of us will have different storage sites distributed around our bodies. Each of us is genetically predisposed to have certain fat storage sites. These sites are your "storage space" where excess fuel is waiting to be used as an energy source. For body fat to be removed, firstly, the fat must be released from the cells into your bloodstream. Once this has been activated, the fatty acids are then used as an energy source burned by the working muscles. In order for fat to be released, adrenaline is secreted. The fat cells have Beta 1 (B1) and Alpha (A 2) receptors. B1 receptors activate the hormone sensitive lipase; this is the enzyme responsible for the breaking down of fat and releasing it into your bloodstream.

> **Did you know?** Abdominal exercises (such as sit ups) have no effect on removing fat from the abdominal areas!

It is a common misconception to think sit-ups will produce that most prized possession – the beautiful flat stomach. There only contribution is how they contribute to a calorie deficit.

Calorie Deficit: The Missing Link to a Flat Stomach

Creating a calorie deficit is a combination of reducing your calories and increasing your activity. This has been scientifically proven as the preferred method of losing weight. As you reduce your calorie consumption, you accelerate your fat loss by adding exercise into the formula.

Cardio training is the fat burning mechanism which removes that layer of fat from your midsection. You must have a balanced eating plan to support a calorie deficit. It boils down to Calories in versus Calories out!!

This programme provides a calorie intake of approximately 1200 calories daily. Latest research supports the theory that this is the most effective calorie range to support weight loss. Some diets suggest a very low calorie intake; but this results in your body being deprived of energy leaving you feeling lethargic and drained.

When you exercise, you accelerate the fat-burning potential by using up to 400 to 500 calories an hour depending on which type of exercise you choose. If resistance training is part of your overall exercise routine, you will develop lean muscle tissue which burns off more calories than soft, flabby metabolically inactive muscle will.

Activity	Calories burned per hour of activity for a 70Kg person.
Aerobics	457
Aerobics (low impact)	352
Ballroom dancing	211
Boxing (competitive)	844
Boxing (punch bag)	422
Carrying an infant	246
Carrying an infant upstairs	352
Circuit training	563
Cycling (leisure to 20 kph)	281 to 563
Football (relaxed to vigorous)	176 to 500
Gardening	281
Golf	317
Hockey	563
Horseback riding	281
Housework	246-281
Judo/Karate/Martial Arts	700
Jumping Rope (skipping)	700
Racquetball/Squash	493-700
Rowing machine	246-600
Rugby	700
Running (normal to vigorous)	563-1000
Sitting in an office chair	106
Swimming	400-700
Tai chi	281
Tennis	493
Walking (slow to very fast)	176-400
Weightlifting	400
Yoga (hatha)	281

As part of the flat stomach 30 day routine, you will incorporate both aerobic and anaerobic training into your weekly schedule. Scientists have carefully researched different weight loss strategies, confirming that a combination of aerobic and anaerobic exercise is the most effective weight loss formula.

Aerobic exercise burns fat by accelerating the fat burning enzymes in your body while improving the functioning of your heart and lungs.

Anaerobic exercise utilises a different energy system which also burns fat but in a different way. Resistance training (lifting weights) is an ideal choice of anaerobic exercise. By incorporating light resistance training you will develop lean metabolically active muscle. This will result in a toned, lean figure.

Protein – The Secret Fat Burner

What role does protein play in fat burning chemistry? Protein has two distinct roles in our weight loss plan:

- Firstly you require protein to build lean muscle tissue. If your body is deprived of protein it will remain shapeless and soft, also it will source energy from breaking down muscle tissue and using it an energy source.
- Secondly, lean muscle tissue built by the protein you consume is metabolically active which supports weight loss. One of the primary functions of your metabolism is to regulate the burning of calories for energy. If your thyroid gland is underactive or overactive it adversely effects the metabolising that takes place in your cells.

What Is Protein?

Protein is a component of very many foods; it is made up of amino acids, which are the building blocks for your bodies tissues and organs. Protein from different food sources has different amino acids. These can be broken down into categories, Non-essential amino acids can be made by your body from an excess of other amino acids in your eating plan. Essential amino acids cannot be made like this and so must be sourced from your eating plan. Protein is required for re-building, growth and repair. Excess protein can also be used as an energy source.

Meat is an excellent source of protein, but there are other alternatives such as non salted nuts, seeds, eggs (organic), soya products, beans, pluses and cheeses. If you do not eat meat, it is crucial to choose a wide variety of proteins which contain essential amino acids. A recent Harvard university study found that "The notion that you could lose weight by cutting out carbohydrates and eating plenty of protein was once tut-tutted by the medical establishment partly because such diets were based on little more than interesting ideas and speculation. In the past two years, head-to-head trials that pitted high-protein, low-carbohydrate diets against low-fat, and high-carbohydrate diets have given them a scientific leg to stand on." These trials show that high-protein, low-carbohydrate diets may work more quickly than low-fat diets, at least in the first six months. After a year or so, though, weight loss is about equal. Compared with a low-fat, high-carbohydrate diet, a higher-protein diet that goes easy on saturated and Trans fats may decrease the amount of triglycerides in the blood, which is also good for the heart.

Why do high-protein, low-carb diets seem to work more quickly than low-fat, high-carbohydrate diets? First, chicken, beef, fish, beans, or other high-protein foods slow the movement of food from the stomach to the intestine. Slower stomach emptying means you feel full for longer and get hungrier later. Second, protein's gentle, steady effect on blood sugar avoids the quick, steep rise in blood sugar and just as quick hunger-bell-ringing fall that occurs after eating a rapidly digested carbohydrate, like white bread or baked potato. Third, the body uses more energy to digest protein than it does to digest fat or carbohydrate.

There's no need, however, to go overboard on protein and eat it to the exclusion of everything else. If you avoid fruits, vegetables and whole grains it means missing out on healthy fibres, vitamins, minerals, and other phytonutrients. It's also important to pay attention to what accompanies protein. Choosing high-protein foods that are low in saturated fat will help the heart even as it helps the waistline.

5

How to Eat: The Eight Super-foods

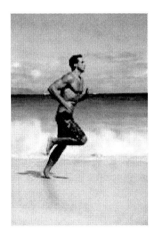

Three Eating Rules for a Flat Stomach

The next thirty days will be a life changing experience for you. You will notice how your energy responds as you ditch the heavily laden processed foods in favour natural alternatives. Mother Nature has supplied you with all the answers; all you have to do is follow the suggested eating plans. There are three Flat stomach rules that you must adhere to if you want to see lasting results.

Rule 1   Stick to between 1200 to 1400 calories a day

Rule 2   No eating after 6.30pm except for something light

Rule 3   Graze! Eat six times per day.

Rule 1: Stick to 1200 calories a day for weight loss

This eating plan provides a calorie intake of around 1200 calories per day. Scientists have carried out careful experiments to confirm that this is the most effective caloric range for removing fat. Contrary to what many think, very low calorie-crash diets of 600 calories per day are not as effective in stimulating weight loss as diets which support the 1200 calorie rule. The participant who on a 600 calories a day diet will be prone to sickness, feel nauseous and lacking in energy. Thus, the caloric allowance suggested by "How to get a flat stomach in 30 days" represents the most effective caloric range for successful weight loss.

Rule 2: No eating after 6.30 pm except for something light

This might be challenging as you may have become accustomed to snacking late at night. In order for any change to take place in your eating regime, it is imperative to <u>not to allow yourself to get hungry</u>. Allow yourself something light around 8pm, like a couple of pieces of fruit, a yogurt. The best food source late at night is protein based as it fills you up. Unsalted nuts or avocado pear is ideal to satisfy your hunger.

Rule 3: Graze - eat six meals a day

It is vital to establish an eating plan which works for you. As a rule if you can envisage sticking to your eating plan for the next five years then you have an achievable eating regime. If you cannot see yourself in five years time still on track, then you must revaluate it. The key is to change your lifestyle choices so you tailor the plan to work for you. If you skip meals, you will become tired and irritable. This is a direct result of your blood sugars falling. By eating every two to two and a half hours you stabilise your blood sugars enabling you to look and feel terrific while losing weight. Snacks should consist of fruit.

The Magic Components

Adding the right combination of super foods will help to speed up your weight loss dramatically. It will also reduce your appetite; relieve digestive problems while targeting the removal of visceral fat. It will also help to correct many years of eating processed and artificial foods. Research has found that people whose eating patterns contain polyunsaturated fats (desirable fats) in place of saturated fats have less visceral fat. Polyunsaturated fats are found in high concentrations in sunflower, corn, and soybean oils, as well as in fish. So what are these super foods?

The Eight Super-foods

1. Vinegar

The Japanese society for Bioscience carried out a range of studies to find a natural way to stop abdominal fat in its tracks. Its findings where surprising; acetic acid which is the main component of vinegar has a lowering effect on your weight and visceral fat. It was concluded that vinegar taken in small doses daily will help to reduce your waistline and more.

2. Oatmeal

Complex carbohydrates, such as grains, fruits and oats take longer for your body to digest which enables you to feel full for longer. They also have a stabilising effect on your blood sugars. This type of complex carbohydrate helps the burning of fat by keeping your insulin levels low, which supports your metabolism in burning calories. In stark contrast, simple carbohydrates such as refined sugary foods create insulin highs and lows which signal a message to your body to store more fat which impedes the efficiency of your metabolism. Research has found oatmeal taken at breakfast is an exceptionally good energy source because it breaks down slowly in your stomach; it encourages your insulin levels to stay low which supports a long lasting energy source. A recent study carried out by the US Navy found that eating a healthy breakfast helped to raise the metabolism by up to 10 percent. Not surprisingly, skipping meals throughout the day slows down the metabolism resulting in your body storing more fat.

3. Green Tea

Green tea contains an important chemical called EGCG which cause your brain and nervous system to run faster, which also helps in the burning of calories. Green tea is also an excellent antioxidant. Green tea has been found to have an overall positive effect on your overall wellbeing and your lungs. The Chinese and Japanese have known this for years and this is why people in this part of the world live longer and are generally healthier than in the west.

4. Nuts (non-salted)

Nuts are an excellent source of protein and fibre and are packed with antioxidants. They may be taken as a snack or mixed with salad or yogurts. One word of warning: they are high in calories so be careful not to have too many. Nuts have an immediate energising effect and also help to lower triglycerides, which contribute to heart disease.

5. Organic Turkey

One the best sources of protein is organic Turkey. It has one of the lowest calorie counts per ounce of any animal protein. As a rule always choose organic, as they are free of pesticides and other chemically enhancing agents.

6. Fruit

Fruit has been hailed as the most perfect food source. It is packed with antioxidants and has the ability to act as a cleansing agent to your cells. Fruit is filled with Glucose, amino acids, minerals and fatty acids. Once fruit is consumed properly (eaten on its own or 30 mins before or after a meal) it becomes alkaline. It has a unique ability to neutralize acid which builds up in your system. Excellent sources of fruit to tackle visceral fat are avocados pears. Smoothies are excellent way to consume fruit or vegetables. Word of caution: do not take in more than 5 pieces of fruit daily as it can lead to an excess of sugars in the blood stream.

7. Organic Yogurt

A study carried out at University of Tennessee found that people who consumed 1200 to 1500 milligrams of calcium daily lost up to twice as much weight as those who consumed less calcium. The lactose in yogurt is fermented by bacteria allowing it to become more digestible as it assists your digestive tract, helping to maintain the correct acidity while improving your immune system. Organic is the only option as it's free of chemical interference.

8. Oily Fish

Oily fish is wonderful source of omega 3 essential fatty acids that support the cleaning of cells in your body. It promotes a clear complexion and helps your brain to function at optimum level. Oily fish contains powerful antioxidants, which can be beneficial in treating asthma, eczema and arthritis. It can reduce the stickiness of your blood, i.e. bad cholesterol, reducing the chances of blood clotting and strokes. Eat steamed or boiled. Fish is also a great source of protein. If you are not a fish lover you may take in capsule form.

Eliminating saturated and Tran's fat, hydrogenated fats from your eating plan is a giant step towards achieving your goal. If you become confused, imagine what it is what you are about to consume is it natural or man made?

By eating a wide selection of different coloured fruits and vegetables daily, you are consuming natural antioxidants. Try spinach, bananas, apples, berries, carrots, water melon etc.

"Eating a diet rich in whole grains while reducing refined carbohydrates changes the glucose and insulin response and makes it easier to mobilize fat stores," according to Penny Kris-Etherton a distinguished professor of nutritional sciences at Penn State University. Ultimately, achieving a flat stomach boils down to taking in fewer calories than you burn. Don't be seduced by the latest guru offering the latest "revolutionary" breakthrough which promises miraculous cures!

6

The Flat Stomach Mindset

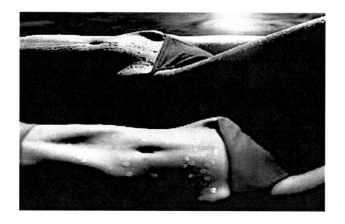

The Battle is Lost or Won in the Mind

The battle for a flat stomach is won or lost in your mind. Years of experience of listening to clients who have tried and failed to lose weight highlight the delicate relationship between mind and the body. Understanding <u>how</u> to get the body and mind working in tandem is the key for your success. Think of how your emotions govern your choice of foods? When you feel low, depleted, tired or angry what do you choose?

The Flat Stomach Formula: MERC

The four pillars for success are:

M Mental Attitude
E Eating Plan
R Resistance Exercise
C Cardiovascular activity

This programme is about customising each part of the MERC formula to meet with your physiological and physical needs. Each segment must work in unison with the other elements for permanent change to take place. Imagine the four wheels of a car, what happens if you remove one wheel? The MERC formula is the very same, you must have all four elements working in harmony.

This chapter is all about the first pillar of the MERC formula: Mental Attitude.

Mental Attitude (*M*ERC)

Lasting change happens within. After reading many stories of men and women who have achieved extraordinary results in their lives I was struck by a common thread running through each biography, their ability to create an unshakable belief in their ability to overcome any obstacle that stood in their path. There is a direct relationship between how well you perform something and your self-image in that area. Your self-image is a blueprint of how you perceive yourself, a reflection of your inner thoughts. You perform as well as you believe you are capable of performing. You cannot surpass on the outside what you believe is on the inside.

> **Did you know?** Your brain function is broken down into two major sections, you're conscious and subconscious.

Your conscious mind is your objective thinking, your rational mind. To illustrate, imagine standing on a bridge and looking down on a train speeding past. Did you notice the carriages racing by? Experts suggest we have up to 60,000 daily thoughts. These carriages resemble thoughts, whizzing through our minds. They react like a conveyer belt, repeating the repetitive thought patterns, over and over, after a prolonged period of constant repetition; these thoughts begin to penetrate your subconscious. Thoughts now become embedded in your subconscious, turning into beliefs; beliefs are a cornerstone of what you know is true. Your self-image is built on a network of beliefs you hold to be true; it is a set of instructions dispatched by your subconscious mind resembling a huge memory bank, which filters out previous similar experiences. The main function of your subconscious mind is to store and retrieve data. It ensures you respond exactly the way it is programmed. Your subconscious enables every belief pattern to be consistent with your self-image. It is pre-programmed. It obeys your belief system and it cannot deviate.

Did you know? Scientists used to believe that humans responded to external stimuli, as they probed to truly understand how we function they discovered that, in fact, we respond to what we believe will happen based on previous experiences.

How do you gain access to your subconscious? Your conscious mind is the gateway! Through constant repetition of words or actions you can enable change. Your conscious mind instructs and your subconscious constructs. Your subconscious mind enables your thought patterns to be consistent with your beliefs.

Conquer Your Subconscious Mind

The subconscious mind operates automatically. It enables your body temperature to regulate at 37ºC, while ensuring you're pulmonary systems function at their correct levels. Your subconscious maintains the correct equilibrium of the cell maintenance and the distribution of the vital minerals and vitamins throughout your body. It keeps highlighting past experiences as a reference point when you decide to change.

Lasting change will only be accomplished once you have established a belief system which is in harmony with your new vision. Change is challenging and you may feel like sliding back to your comfort zone.

The law of the subconscious mind states that whatever you believe is true will be accepted by your subconscious mind and it will go about bringing into reality what you have instructed to be true. Your subconscious is your central processing facility. Words become actions, pictures you hold are drawn to you, you become a magnet for your dominate thoughts. Once you have brought into your reality a belief, this reconfirms your belief, lodging it deeper into your subconscious mind. The biggest hurdle is to overcome self limiting beliefs. Whatever you believe, it will become your reality through constant repetition, and you will behave, talk and interact in a manner consistent with your core beliefs.

Believing in you is paramount for change. Having the self-confidence to pursue your quest for a flat stomach and believing you can is your responsibility.

The Law of Cause and Effect

This law states that for every effect in your life there is a specific cause. Goals are causes, health and wellbeing are effects. Goals begin as thoughts or causes and manifest themselves as effects. This law also states that everything happens for a reason, there are no accidents. We live in an orderly universe governed by strict laws, and understanding this is central to every law or principle. The law of cause and effect states that there are very specific reasons for creating any effect in your life. If you wish to create more of a particular effect, trace it back to the causes and repeat the causes. If you wish to terminate a particular effect, trace it back to its cause and eliminate it. Insanity was once described as doing the same things in the same way and expecting to get different results. The most important thing to remember about this law is for weight loss is that thoughts are causes and body shape is the effects.

The solution must treat the cause; People who have achieved their ideal weight are using the law of cause and effect, whether consciously or unconsciously. They do not allow any contradictory thoughts to take root in their minds. Their predominant thoughts are on what effect their actions will cause. They focus on the end result, eliminating any negative behaviour. Nothing comes into existence from the outside; it is the manifestation of your dominant thought patterns and emotions which produce the causes and effects in your life.

Your solution must have all the ingredients, and it is an amalgamation of both body and mind. Before you discover the formula, you must understand why you gained weight? What physiological factors contributed to your weight gain?

Latest research from America shows that your brain is a goal-searching mechanism. Go somewhere that you will not be disturbed, close your eyes, and banish any thoughts or worries. Allow yourself to completely relax. Once you have established feeling relaxed, I want to think what do you really want? Get a picture of what you really want deep down. If possible get a photo and use this as a trigger. In order to realise a goal, it must meet three specific requirements.

1. It must be specific—go into as much detail as possible, how you will look? How you will feel? What kind of clothes will you wear?
2. It must have a deadline: "I will be X Kg by the 21st of May". This gives clarity and focus.
3. It must be in writing. Unless it is written down; it will remain only a distant dream. By writing it down, you are declaring it.

The Ultimate Flat Stomach Goal Setting Formula

Step 1: Be inspired to take action

Fix in your mind the exact goal that you desire. Be definite as to what you want. What do you really want? Sit down and write it out. If you are unsure about your goal you are sending out mixed signals which bring about mixed responses. Now for the first time in your life maybe, identify what you really want. This is the first step in the process. Then establish what your unique motivating factor is? Find that one image which sends shivers through your body with excitement. Once you have firmly established the end goal and believe you can achieve it, you have created a defining moment in your life.

Step 2: What you will give in return?

Determine exactly what you are going to give in return. What service will you provide to justify achieving your goal?

Step 3: Establish a definite date & hard work

There is no avoiding this. No pills or magic potions can replace hard work. It has been often said that the two of the most powerful words in the English language are discipline and regret. It takes discipline and effort, but the rewards are indescribable. Imagine the pride you will feel when you accomplish your goal. Write down your goal, a deadline and place it where you can see daily. Visualise daily your desired outcome. The trick is to deeply embed your goal in your subconscious mind. This is done by constant repetition of your desired outcome.

Step 4: Create a definite plan

You must know how you will achieve your goal. The skills and knowledge which will provide the results you want. Find a role model, someone who has achieved what you want. Identify their structure and replicate each step. Use this book as your role model for losing weight.

Step 5: Write out a clear, concise statement of achieving your goal

Write the date by which you will achieve your goal followed by a definite plan of action. Describe your plan of action in detail. Break down your goal into sizeable chunks, example monthly goal followed by a weekly goals followed by a daily goals.

Step 6: Self belief & read out your statement

Read out aloud your statement, twice daily, just before retiring at night and once when you arise in the morning. **Self-belief** is the defining element which catapults your dreams into reality, separating you from your peers. By believing in yourself it will instil the necessary confidence and enthusiasm to create your objective. All of your power to create the life you want is available to you right now.

The trigger to your success is the ability to imprint your desired image on your subconscious mind. This is done by constant repetition of affirmations through your conscious mind. Your subconscious mind must photograph the desired result; this forms a new internal dialogue, where the subconscious brings about this new image. Imagine your subconscious as a computer, installing a new programme. This is the key to unlocking the door. This picture gives you clarity, motivation and focus. Most goals fall into the category of wishful thinking; they are wishes, remaining in the conscious mind. Each journey is a series of small steps taken in the right direction. Regardless of your wishes, they will not happen until you have created a clear vision of the final outcome and by running this image over and over knowing that every step you take is taking you one step closer to your vision. Every goal has a format. It is a question of mapping out what guidelines they follow.

Cancer of the Soul

Negativity is a cancer which seeps into every orifice of your body, it is a disease spreading its tentacles into every nook and cranny of your emotional & physical wellbeing, it saps your enthusiasm and immobilises change while keeping you firmly entrenched in your comfort zone. Remember that you control your conscious thought patterns. Thought are objects! Positive or negative, repeated thoughts become your reality. Truly your mind can be your greatest asset or greatest liability.

Have you ever wondered what helps you to achieve that flat stomach? Is it eating less, changing habits or exercising? It is the motivation which is the driving force behind lasting change. Adopting the correct mind set is the crucial. To truly believe you can achieve your goal is the first rule of achieving a flat stomach in 30 days.

"How do I stop my negative thoughts?" - is a question often asked. There is a simple answer, concentrate only on positive thoughts. Positive thought patterns will counteract negative impulses. By focusing on your fears, you literally attract them into your life. They can never disappear because you are focusing on them. The truth is always easy. To stop negative thoughts, just sow positive thoughts! By deliberately concentrating on the positive outcome you attract this response into your life. You will wipe out all opposing or negative thoughts. Focusing on what you want and not on what you don't want to happen will ensure a positive outcome. Try for one day to only focus on positive thoughts! Don't let any negativity set in. You will be very surprised at the results!

As another exercise: try smiling more! Force yourself to smile even when you don't feel like it. Don't just do a weak smile – you need to do a full, teeth exposed, Hollywood smile. Recent research has shown that the facial muscles involved in smiling, when contracted, trigger the brain to release happy hormones making you feel instantly happier and more positive. Try it and see for yourself!

Carrot and Stick Motivation

The carrot motivation is about keeping your goal ahead of you. Maybe it is an upcoming wedding or that long awaited vacation. These future events are the vocal point to change.

Carrot motivation
- Insert a photo of your final goal in your purse.
- Look at it at least once a day
- Image yourself in that swimsuit, dress or pair of jeans.
- Count the days on your calendar for the big day.
- Set three small goals daily that you must achieve.
- Set weekly goals.

Stick motivation
- Insert a photo of when you felt overweight.
- Hang up a pair of jeans or dress you could not fit into.
- Track your progress weekly.
- Measure yourself before you begin the programme.
- Reassess your weekly progress.

Which works for you? The most effective approach is usually a blending of both: seeing how you will look, while remembering how you felt when you were overweight.

Success Leaves Footprints for You

One of the most positive things about the internet is the abundance of knowledge which you have access to instantly. Someone has already achieved exactly what you want. They have left a trail of footprints to your goal. For virtually everything you want to do, there are courses and books on how to do it. When you take advantage of this information, you will discover that all you have to do is follow their trail, use their system, personalising it for your needs.

Searching for footprints

1. Find a role model and seek their help, unravel their dominant thought patterns.
2. Search the internet, books and courses for information which you can adapt to your requirements.
3. Identify exactly what you want, and seek local activities which you can learn from.

7

The Flat Stomach Action Plan

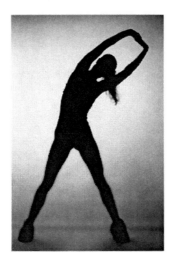

Action is What Unites Vision with Success

The greatest secret in the world is also the greatest secret to success. It is revealed in the old saying: *take action*! You may have a wonderful vision, great ideas, brilliant strategies, etc. but it all counts for nothing unless you create a forward momentum for taking action. Action creates results, without taking action there are no results. Action is what unites vision and results. Action begins by gathering the correct knowledge or gaining the skills required to make your vision happen. Your vision gives clarity and a sense of direction to your life. Without goals or action, your vision will remain a figment of your imagination. You <u>must</u> take action and you must have a strategy. A strategy is basically a road map of how to get where you want to go. You've probably heard the phrase "take action" countless times in your lifetime but how many times have you put it into practice? It is the most valuable thing you can do in any endeavour.

Acquiring the proper knowledge or learning new skills will take time. If you are reading this book then I am pretty sure that your goal is to obtain a flat stomach. In order to reach this achievement, you must first acquire the proper knowledge otherwise your attempts will be fruitless. Regardless of what action you take, you must understand <u>how</u> to get a flat stomach. Secondly, you must take the <u>appropriate steps</u> to make it happen.

Individuals who have achieved greatness in their lives do something that 99% of people do not do: they take immediate, informed action. Wishing and dreaming will not change your life but action will. Decisions are prerequisite for your success; it defines where you are and where you are going. The most powerful way to change your life is by taking consistent actions but what precedes actions? <u>Decisions</u>!

I <u>Will</u> Act Now!

Procrastination must be avoided at all costs. Stop dreaming and start doing. That pretty sums up how to achieve success!

> "Genius is made up of 99% perspiration and 1% inspiration."
>
> **Thomas Edison**

It is remarkable how real inspirational stories can transform our lives, giving us the impetus to take action. It is profound to read the stories of brave individuals who have overcome insurmountable obstacles in order to reach their dream. There are many stories which provoke such admiration as individuals battled to succeed despite facing racial, economic, physical, emotional and social disadvantages. They achieved what many would deem impossible due to their discipline, work ethic and self-belief.

To find the real secret of such stories, we must look beneath the surface to understand what actions they took to make their vision come alive. It becomes apparent in most cases that these extraordinary individuals were driven by an insatiable hunger for success and were prepared to do everything in their power to make it happen; in short they wanted it more than anyone else.

Plenty of remarkable stories have been handed down through the years concerning the successes of people in the political arena, the world of sports and cultural icons form the world of film and arts. A perfect illustration is Lance Armstrong who won the toughest cycling race in the world, Tour De France no less than seven times. Bear in mind, he battled a deadly form of cancer and yet still managed to succeed. He once said: "Winning is about heart, not just legs. It's got to be in the right place." The legendary basket ball player Michael Jordan failed to make it on to the basketball team on his first year, yet he ended up becoming perhaps the greatest basketball player of all time. These are real inspirational heroes who achieved their dream of world domination in their particular field due to their courage and the actions they took. They didn't wake up one day and become champions. They worked harder than anybody else and never gave up on their dream.

You may a wonderful hopes, ideas, brilliant strategies but it all counts for nothing unless you create a forward momentum for taking action. Action creates results, without taking action there are no results.

Seeing What you Want and Making it Happen

Visualization is the art of seeing in your mind's eye a picture of exactly what you want; it is possibly the most underused success tool at your disposal. It powerfully accelerates the interaction of your subconscious mind.
1. Visualization activates the sensory tools of your subconscious mind.
2. Visualization heightens the desire of your goal, allowing you to notice how you will feel both mentally and physically.
3. Visualization will enable you to truly believe you can create your desired outcome.

The Magic of Believing

Sports coaches searched for generations to identify why certain players excelled and others with similar talents did not. How can one person create extraordinary achievements and others fall by the wayside? After much research, neuropsychologists have found that we become conditioned to believe in certain outcomes. This magical belief generates the passion which propels you to push beyond endurance because you truly believe you are going to achieve your goal. It is that indescribable quality which separates winners from losers. Our brain has become conditioned to expect a certain response, we get what we really <u>believe</u> will happen. One of the powerful techniques is to behave as if the desired outcome has happened. By behaving in a manner consistent with the inner image, your outer behaviour will create the inner experience. It will allow you to adopt the correct mind set. Recent research has compounded what was originally believed: when your brain is seeing an activity being completed it cannot distinguish between *seeing* it being accomplished and *actually* accomplishing it.

Visualization focuses your attention. Many sports physiologists are insisting that athletes visualize the desired outcome. Peak performance experts are using visualization as a part of their performance enhancing techniques.

The Art of Visualizing a Flat Stomach

Enter the magical and powerful world of visualization, the art of imagining your desired goal and what it will feel like, this instils the necessary energy to pursue your objective.

How to visualize? When you visualize your goals as already have been achieved it creates a belief pattern in your subconscious mind. This in turn creates "structural tension" where your reality and your projected goal are in the process of becoming united. Your subconscious mind tries to resolve the process by bringing in to your reality your vision. Find a place you can relax and will be undisturbed. Close your eyes and see your objective having been completed.

Visualize it in detail: Andre Agassi the famous tennis player is said to have visualized the T-shirt he would be wearing when he won the Wimbledon tennis tournament! He also visualized the sounds of people cheering for him and the feeling he would get when he touched the cup. In short you need to visualize the slightest details in order to intensify the experience.

Visualize the performance by carefully selecting the most effective strategies and belief patterns which support your best possible performance. When you produced your best results previously, what where the key components responsible for this? What did you feel? What did you believe? How where you empowered to take action? What motivated you? What image did you use? By duplicating the most effective mental and physical strategies it will enable you to reproduce the same results.

Visualize over & over: When you visualize your goals as already complete every day, it creates conflict in your subconscious mind between what your reality is and what you are visualizing. Your subconscious mind will resolve the difference by bringing into your reality the picture you hold as your new reality.

Visualize your most powerful image: select your most powerful image. This image generates the necessary motivation to bring about your reality.

Visualize am & pm: One of the most striking findings recently discovered suggests that to visualize just before going to sleep and upon awaking is the most effective time frame which encourages the image to linger in the subconscious mind.

The art of visualization is quite simple. Begin by selecting a quiet place where you will not be disturbed. Simply close your eyes and see your goal as if it was accomplished. If your objective is to have a flat stomach, fill in as many details as possible. Make the image as clear as possible, write down your objective and goal. Visualize daily your desired outcome. Then, every morning when you wake and each night just before you go to sleep, picture your outcome if it has already happened. Re-create the end result as if it has been already completed.

Another tip is to put a photo in your purse or wallet. It will constantly remind you of your final destination. Psychologists suggest this is the most powerful way to reinforce and propel you towards your goal. Emotions are the most powerful way of propelling your reality towards your vision.

Visualization Really Works!!

Wimbledon champion Andre Agassi describes how he visualized his success. "I have already won Wimbledon at least 10,000 times before." People first laughed because they believed he was joking but when Andre explained that he had visualized himself winning the tournament thousands of times people realized the power of visualization.

Visualization is a very powerful tool that can help you reach your goals if you used it correctly. Lots of people confuse visualization with day dreaming, while the second is just a helpless attempt a desperate person makes to in order feel good about themselves, the first is a way that motivates the mind and ignites the passion towards reaching a certain goal. If you never have managed to taste the feeling you are going to experience when you finally achieve your goal, then you will never be truly motivated to pursue it. Why would you? What is going to sustain you through the months as you strive to achieve your goal if you have no idea of what it will feel like when you finally arrive?

Just Do It!

Action is what unites dreams with reality. There are two types of people, one who sits around thinking of doing it and the other is the person who does it! Taking decisive steps with strategic planning is a trigger which propels you to success. Whether it's developing a plan of action or making a series of small daily changes, nothing will be accomplished until you just do it! Becoming too analytical or over planning is often a cop out. I'll say it again: there are two types of people, one who sit around waiting for all of the cosmic elements to be aligned correctly before they venture into the unknown or the other type of people who just go and do it! Action is what unites every success.

I Will Take Action Today!

The Power of Momentum

Every great journey is a series of small steps taken in the right direction. Never stray from the path! Regardless of how insignificant the steps may seem, small changes done on a daily basis will create a significant change over time. The momentum of your actions will carry you towards your chosen target. Play tricks with your mind by rewarding yourself daily for having completed your daily tasks, build in 20 minutes a day for rewarding yourself. Change your exercise regime and do what you want to do today! If it is sunny, go for a power walk outside. Enjoy the process and reward yourself. This positive activity has a much stronger physiological effect because you know you are steadily moving towards your goal. Hitting your daily targets gives you the confidence to pursue your final goal; you know it is only a matter of time before you arrive at your final destination. Enjoy the journey. Keep the mind fresh, change routines and eating plans daily to keep it fresh.

The Daily To-do-List

What actions must I do today? List three specific goals every day, include them in a journal.

1. Today I will.....

2. Today I will......

3. Today I will.....

Write out each morning three objectives which must be completed by the end of the day, and tick them off before you go bed. Learn to prioritise by identifying what you are struggling with. Your biggest challenge should be your number one goal which must be completed. This gives clarity and focus to your day. Remember, there is almost always a person who has achieved precisely what you want, Select a role model; identify their dominant thought patterns and behaviours and try to follow their tracks.

Create One Ground-breaking Goal

Divide every aspect of your vision into smaller goals; also create one major goal that will represent a gigantic leap for you. Once you have set your goal and deadline, work backwards, breaking your goal into monthly, weekly and daily targets. Create that milestone, the first part of the journey. This sets in train a series of steps which is called the confidence cycle. It enables you to believe you can achieve your ultimate goal. The first milestone could be to lose 2 pounds within 6 days! This is a quantum leap in your progression, both physically and physiologically. The achievement of that one step will set in motion a chain of positive events for the successful completion of your ultimate goal. What is your milestone? Take small steps!

The next step on your journey is to activate the powers of your subconscious mind by reading your goals twice a day, last thing at night and first thing in the morning. Closing your eyes and seeing your goal accomplished. Notice how you look? How you feel? The confidence of knowing you succeeded. This ritual will stoke the fires of your subconscious as its focuses on bringing this goal into reality. Experts call this the "structural tension" where your subconscious mind closes the gap between the projected image and your reality.

Fears, Diversions and Cul-De-Sacs

It is important to note that as soon as you decide on a new plan, three obstacles may appear. Forewarned is forearmed!! Do not be discouraged if you meet these unwelcome visitors!!

1. Fear

Your old beliefs may manifest. These feelings are of failure, rejection and scorn. What will people say? Will they laugh at me? What happens if this does not work? You may try to shield yourself physiologically by not really attempting the challenge. These negative thought patterns are common. Fear destroys our dreams, keeping us chained to a life of mediocrity. This fear of failure is a conditioned survival technique we have learnt. These fears are usually at the upper and lower limits of our comfort zone. The process of dismantling these fears begins with positive affirmations about you. This repeated thought pattern overrides fears. Setting daily goals that you achieve increase your self confidence. Everything goes back to your self-image, how you perceive yourself, that blueprint which has being programmed into your subconscious is the answer.

2. Diversions

You may experience temporary setbacks, everything may not go exactly as planned; these are merely obstacles you must deal with. In truth very little in life goes exactly to plan so don't let it divert you from your ultimate goal.

3. Cul-de-sacs

Cul-de-sacs (or dead-ends) are another form of temporary setbacks; it is common to encounter challenges along the path to change. Things may not go as smoothly as planned. This is part of the challenge, how will you navigate successfully through these blips? Don't get discouraged. These are pitfalls. Learn to handle these as merely a natural part of your progression. Once you have overcome these obstacles, it instils a scene of pride as you realise your full potential.

Small Steps to Lasting Change

At times, goals may be overwhelming. Stepping back, looking at the mountain ahead, may be daunting. Everyone has their own unique challenges. Breaking larger goals down into weekly and daily tasks make the process more accessible.

STEP 2

THE PROGRAMME

8

The Flat Stomach in 30 Days Eating Plan

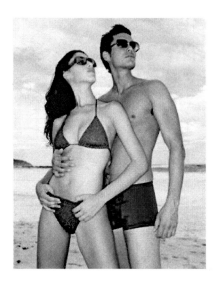

Change Your Life and Never Look Back

Here comes exactly what you need to start right now to losing weight, it is do-able and you can mould it to fit your lifestyle. The complete eating plan is broken down into 5 categories. Low GI fruit, natural starches, protein, vegetables and dairy products. The key details are:

1. Consume three servings of 100g (4oz) protein choices per day. Choose from: white meat, red meat (twice per week), fish, eggs, low fat cheese, goat's cheese, and non salted nuts.

2. Natural starches have a stabilising effect on your blood sugar, allowing you to feel energised for long periods. Take in two portions of low GI starches, brown rice, whole meal bread, pasta or lentils per day.

3. Dairy products are full of calcium which supports bone development. Allow for two to three portions of low fat

organic dairy products, yogurt, skimmed milk or soya milk per day.

4. Fruit, it is full of natural antioxidants, vitamins and minerals, but can contain high levels of fructose, choose low GI fruits. Good choices are Apples, oranges, avocado, pears, melons and bananas.

5. Vegetables which are low GI can be consumed in large quantities as they are low in calories and rich in vitamins, minerals and other nutrients.

Clean Eating

Replace toxic food with clean foods. To simplify, chose foods which have not been tampered with. Choose:
- Foods which have not changed from their original state.
- Foods which are not "fat free" or "lite"
- Foods which have no added salt or flavouring.
- Foods which do not last for months!!
- Foods that do not have sugar as their main ingredient.
- Foods that do not leave you feeling bloated!!
- Foods which are not manmade.

Shopping List

This is a Guide that will give you an idea of the types of food you will need to stock up your fridge/cupboards with.

1.   Fruit, Vegetables and Seeds

Broccoli	Mango
Carrots	Apples
Onions/Garlic (for cooking)	Bananas
Peppers	Berries – various
Mange tout	Plums
Green Beans	Kiwi
Courgettes	Pineapple
Aubergine	Carrot /Apple /Orange juice (fresh)
Tomatoes	Melon
Cucumber	Flaxseed or Linseed
Salad leaves/lettuce	Sesame seeds
Mushrooms	Sunflower seeds
	Pumpkin seeds

2.   General

Porridge Oats
Brazil Nuts
Milk or Soya milk (Low fat)
Olives
Chick peas / mixed beans (Naked
Bean Company is ideal)

Fresh fish:
Mackerel, salmon, herring, trout
are best) cod, haddock, whiting,
lemon sole etc are also excellent.
Shell fish (in moderation)

Chicken
Turkey
Tofu
Humus
Eggs
Tuna
Goats cheese (1st choice) 0r Feta
/ Cottage
Natural organic yoghurt
Water Biscuits or Nairn's Oat
cakes
Water or Water filter jug
Green Tea / herbal teas

3.   In moderation

Lean Meat
Cambridge's Brown Bread
Brown Rice
Baking Potatoes
Avocado
Pine nuts (for salads etc)

30 Days Flat Stomach Eating Plan (MERC)

Breakfast

Choose one of the following
- Three pieces of fruit with organic yogurt mixed through if required
- Oatmeal made of skimmed milk with berries mixed through
- Fruit smoothies
- Omelette with tomato and mushrooms

Also have
- 2 glasses of spring water and one cup of green tea

11am
- Banana or one piece of fruit of your choosing

Lunch
Choose one of the following
- Grilled fish with a green salad, vinegar
- Goats cheese with a salad of your choosing
- Bowl of fresh vegetable soup with a slice of brown wholemeal bread
- Chicken salad

Also have
- Olive oil dressing
- 2 glasses of water
- Organic yoghurt of your choice

4pm
- Red apple

Dinner
Choose a 170g (6oz) portion of one of the following
- Beef
- Fish
- Poultry

Also have two handfuls of fresh vegetables:
- Green beans
- Broccoli
- Peppers
- Spinach
- Peas
- Carrots

8 pm
Choose from one of the following
- Crisp bread with some low fat cheese
- Organic yoghurt with some non salted cashew nuts mixed in
- A carrot and apple smoothie
- A slice of melon

Now that you know exactly what to eat you should follow the above eating plan exactly as it is given above!

Things that you MUST do every day:

- Allow 2 units of carbohydrate per day along with the above food plan (one unit is a cup size).
- Take in two units of dairy products per day
- Consume 3 to 5 pieces of fruit per day.
- Drink 2 litres of water per day
- Take green vegetables daily
- Take one cup of green tea per day
- Take some form of protein at night if possible.
- Become sugar & salt free
- Stop the stimulants (coffee, cola drinks, etc)
- Remove processed and convenience food from your eating plan.
- Limit alcohol to 3 units per week – if you do drink then organic red wine is preferable.
- Eat avocado pears
- Consume vinegar
- Take in non salted nuts

Things that you must NOT do every day:

- Do not eat large meals after 6.30pm
- Do not eat take away food
- Do not drink more than one cup of coffee per day
- Do not eat possessed or frozen foods
- Do not eat junk food
- Do not drink more than 4 units of alcohol per week.
- Do not eat red meat more than twice per week.

A healthy balanced plan is crucial to be healthy. Certain fad diets, for example, claim that omitting carbohydrates from your overall eating plan will allow you to lose weight. What these fad diets do not tell you, however, is that most of the weight is actually fluid retention! Many of these high profile diets claim scientific facts as the basis for losing weight, what they do not tell you is what you are actually doing to your body. These days, people in general consume far too much processed protein. Growth hormones and chemical pesticides are given to most animals and what do you think happens to us when we consume this meat? Researchers have uncovered an array of health problems associated with eating this type of meat. The key is to try to eat organic food as this is free of chemical interference.

Did you know?

If you want to see results without making a big effort, getting a pet could be the way to go. Multiple research studies have shown that pet owners have improved physical and mental health, including lowered blood pressure, better ability to cope with adverse life effects, and lowered stress levels. For those who need encouragement to up their fitness levels, getting a pet dog may also provide you with that push you need to get out and get active.

For most people who have ever tried to lose weight, the thought of going on a diet congers up many unsavoury images. The lists of forbidden foods, the willpower required, feeling rotten, low energy levels etc. which is ultimately followed by getting to the finish line and then retuning to your normal eating patterns. Disaster is lurking just around the corner. Those dreaded pounds which were so difficult to remove reappear in no time. For you to truly succeed, you must readjust your understanding of diet and incorporate healthy lifestyle choices. "How to Get a Flat Stomach in 30 Days" is a way of life, it is a way readjusting to a more health conscious way of living. It is not there to restrict but to enhance your life. This book promises to give you a flat stomach in 30 days; it will also reduce the risk of contacting any of the deadly diseases associated with visceral fat. Overwhelming research has supported the finding that particular foods will increase or decrease the levels of visceral fat present in your body.

Knowing full well that this book would have to compete with numerous books offering weight loss etc, it was vital that "How to Get a Flat Stomach in 30 days" would need something unique that no other book could offer. Firstly, this book offers the definite eating plan which I have just shown you. This plan has been scientifically proven as the ultimate weight loss package. There are no fads and no gimmicks, if you follow the eating plan exactly as I have just shown you then you <u>will</u> lose weight! This is the <u>perfect eating plan</u>! Why? Well it is perfect because it allows you to tailor it to suit your lifestyle. Go back and look at the eating plan and see how there are <u>options</u> for each meal. You don't like fish? No problem, pick from one of the other choices given.

Daily Eating Plan Tracker
This will allow you monitor your daily intake. It is invaluable to track your daily progress. Photocopy this page, or rewrite it in your diary or journal, and keep a record of what you ate:

Breakfast
- Water consumption:
- Protein:
- Carbohydrates:

Mid-morning snack:

Lunch
- Water consumption
- Protein:
- Carbohydrates:

Mid-Afternoon snack: Fruit

Dinner
- Protein:
- Carbohydrates:

Supper
- Protein:
- Carbohydrates:

Total Daily Units:
Water: Fat: Fruit: Vegetables:

This book uses the MERC formula as its central philosophy. The MERC formula is all about changing your lifestyle and it makes doing this as easy as possible by giving you choices rather than dictating to you. The eating plan I have given you asks you to eat six meals a day not to skip meals or eat less at each meal. The truth is that skipping meals can cause you to gain weight because it slows down your metabolism and destabilizes your blood sugars. In fact, people who skip meals tend to be heavier that those who eat regularly. This may be due to the fact that individuals who skip meals tend to overeat and also eat at the wrong times. A more sensible approach is to reduce your calories and avoid long fasting period's and that is what I have shown you in the eating plan.

Handy Calorie Counter:
You should use the eating plan above and try to stay within 1200 calories per day.

Potato: 2 medium sized potatoes = 150 calories
Oatmeal: regular sized portion = 140 calories
Chicken: regular portion = 250
Steak: medium size = 350 calories
Glass of milk: medium size = 90 calories
Apple: 60 to 80 calories
Banana: 90 to 100 calories
Egg: 96 calories
1 slice of brown bread = 70 calories
1 slice of normal bread = 70 calories
1 slice of batch bread = 140 calories
Yogurt: small pot = 100 calories
Wine: one glass (125ml) = 150 calories
Vegetables: medium size portion = 60 calories
Cheese: 2 small portions of low fat cheese = 100 calories
Beans: medium size portion = 40 calories
Wrap: medium size = 50 calories

Note: In most cases, a medium sized portion is approximately ½ the size of your palm.

9

The Flat Stomach Workout

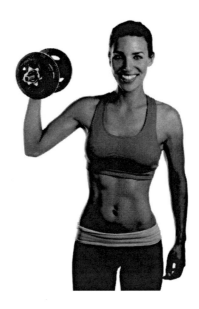

Science Supports Exercise over Diet Alone!

A recent study from the USA has shown that exercise can get the best weight loss results. Why is that? Even though both diet and exercise are equally effective for losing pounds, there is nevertheless a significant advantage to exercise in that you get fitter in the process. "Weight loss through exercise provides greater benefits because it increases your capacity to perform physical activity while diet-induced weight loss does not provide such a benefit," according to the lead researcher, Dr. Edward Weiss at Saint Louis University. For the study, researchers recruited 34 volunteers: 18 dieted while 16 engaged in moderate exercise such as a brisk walk for an hour, six times a week. After one year, both groups had lost about the same amount of weight - about 10 per cent of their body weight, which is considered healthy weight loss. But there was a marked difference in fitness levels:

- The exercises <u>maintained</u> their strength and muscle mass and <u>increased</u> their aerobic capacity.
- The dieters <u>lost</u> muscle mass, <u>lost</u> strength and <u>lost</u> aerobic capacity.

Dieting alone is bad news for effective weight loss in the long run because the muscles of dieters actually became "de-conditioned" because they are now carrying around a lighter load. "Once a person loses weight, his or her muscles don't have to work as hard at every day movements, such as rising from a chair, walking up steps or getting out of a car", explains Dr. Weiss. Dr. Weiss has cautioned that dieting can be important for losing extra pounds in the first place, but what is most important is maintaining the new lower weight. "If push comes to shove and someone wanted to know if they should diet or exercise to lose weight, I would suggest exercise, provided they are willing to put in the extra time and effort and not offset the gains they make by eating more," commented Dr. Weiss when his groundbreaking study was released

Lose the Bulge!

Now that you understand the basics of balanced nutrition, you're ready to do some major re-shaping, I know from experience how difficult it can be to fit in an exercise routine into your busy life. That is why the following routines can be adapted to suit your schedule. I know firsthand the benefits of aerobic exercise and what resistance training can do to enhance your figure and self-confidence, as well as minimising the risk of disease. It is vital that *"How to Get a Flat Stomach in 30 days"* should include an exercise plan that can be customised to fit your schedule. Remember that the eating plan is designed to provide a flat stomach in 30 days; I know from personal experience spanning over two decades that aerobic exercise and resistance training will reshape your figure and boost your energy levels as well as strengthening bone and muscle mass. This exercise routine will reshape your figure: your abdominals, thighs, hips and also remodel your arms and chest. The exercising routines will accelerate your results dramatically. This exercise format is broken down into three distinct "Zones".

The Three Exercise "Zones"

Zone 1: Abdominals.
Zone 2: Fitness.
Zone 3: Tonality.

Each zone works in tandem with the other, accentuating your tonality while improving your fitness. The chest, thighs, butt and triceps will be reconstructed, removing excess weight and replacing it with lean muscle tissue. With the flat stomach workout, you will concentrate on each zone, focusing on selective exercises which will allow maximum results in the shortest time frame. By employing these techniques, you choose which specific areas need to be highlighted. "Spot reduction" is accomplished by using light resistance training to target stubborn areas. The overall effect is a remodelled figure. There is an ongoing debate about spot reduction. One side suggest it is impossible to select areas at will, while the other side suggest it is possible. There are merits in both sides of the argument. By following the eating plan as suggested and combine it with exercise plan outlined, you can target specific areas by working them 3 times per week with light weights. Blood circulated through soft muscle tissues is slow. When you exercise it increases the blood flow to the muscle which promotes the release of fat which is stored in these pockets. The workouts will subtract inches of fat while replacing it with lean muscle tissue.

Zone 1: The Abdominals (Stomach Area)

Your abdominals are your "core" muscle group, all movement stems from this focal point. Luckily, this area responds quickly and in particular when you perform a combination of light resistance training and aerobic training. The key is to do plenty of aerobic work and finish with core and abdominal exercises. Performing the correct abdominal exercises will ensure a lean, firm stomach. The following exercises are the most effective. A strong, firm mid-section will improve your posture and help to prevent lower back problems. The best abdominal exercises are surprisingly easy to do. A recent study carried out to find the best tummy flattening exercises by The Biomechanics Lab at

San Diego State University found that the top abdominal exercises are:

1. Bicycle Crunch Exercise

How to Do it
- Lie flat on the floor with your lower back pressed to the ground.
- Put your hands beside your head.
- Bring your knees up to about a 45-degree angle and slowly go through a bicycle pedal motion.
- Touch your left elbow to your right knee, then your right elbow to your left knee.
- Breathe evenly throughout the exercise.
- Repeat until you cannot do any more

2. Crunch on an Exercise Ball

How to do it
- Sit on the exercise ball with your feet flat on the floor.
- Let the ball roll back slowly and lie back until your thighs and torso are parallel with the floor.
- Contract your abdominals (tummy muscles) raising your torso to no more than 45 degrees.
- Repeat until your stomach muscles are so tired that they cannot do any more.
- To work the oblique muscles (side of the tummy) make the exercise less stable by moving your feet closer together.

3. Vertical Leg Crunch Abdominal Exercise

How to Do it
- Lie on your back and extend the legs up with knees slightly bent.
- Contract your abs and rise up until your shoulder blades leave the floor.
- Keep your chin up; don't pull on your neck.
- Keep your legs in a fixed position.
- Lift your torso toward your knees.
- Lower and repeat for 12-16 repetitions.

Zone 2: Fitness

For removing body fat, I recommend that you perform cardiovascular work in two different ways. The first method is long steady distances and the second method is Interval training. In the *"How to Get a Flat Stomach in 30 Days"* plan, you will alternate between two different heart rates in the same session and create the aerobic wave. This combination of long slow pace combined with interval training makes your body burn fat in the most efficient way. This is achieved by the raising of your basal metabolic rate (BMR) which is the rate at which you burn calories when you are resting. It is crucial to destroy the excess weight around the mid section by using two weapons: weapon number one being the eating plan and weapon number two is cardiovascular work. It is also incorrect to suggest that cardiovascular activity alone will burn off the fat from your mid section. If there is one crucial element for achieving a flat stomach it must be your eating plan. This is of absolute paramount importance. The abdominal area is known as "Lipolytically active". This means your midsection responds favourably to aerobic exercise. Engaging in aerobic exercise, adrenalin is released to increase the fatty acid content in your blood stream so fuel can be sourced. Fat cells respond quickly to adrenaline, resulting in fatty cells being disposed of. Recent studies carried out found that aerobic exercise is particularly effective in burning away unwanted storage fat from the abdominal areas.

Zone 3: Tonality

Your glutes (muscles in the bottom) thighs and hips will respond immediately to cardiovascular activity. By reshaping your lower body, it will give you that toned look, accentuating your upper body while minimising your waist. Your bum and thighs may have become un-shapely due to a lack of exercise but help is at hand. The following exercise routines will give you that slimmer profile by tightening and toning the above areas. Plus, for ladies, you'll improve, define and accentuate your cleavage and, if like most women, you dislike the size of your thighs (and are sick of trying to camouflage their size with baggy pants), then don't despair: this exercise routine will help to trim your thighs from large to slim.

The 3 pillars of the flat stomach workout

1. Aerobic exercise - which burns away fat deposit sites and increases your fitness levels.
2. Resistance training - which sculpts and reshapes your body and promotes the burning of calories up to 24 hours after you have exercised. It also strengthens your bone density and has many anti-aging benefits.
3. Core work - this strengthens your abdominal area while improving your posture and strengthens your lower back.

The winning combination: for best results, I recommend using both aerobic exercise and resistance training. As your body slowly transforms to a leaner, toned athletic physic, you will look and feel better within weeks.

The Benefits of Aerobic exercise

- Burns body fat.
- Improves the efficiency of calorie burning.
- Reduces inches from your stomach.
- Improves your fitness levels.
- Improves your over all wellness.

Accelerating Fat Loss with Aerobic Work

Aerobic exercise includes a range of activities which will increase your heart rate leaving you slightly breathless. Power walking, swimming, jogging or cycling fall within the aerobic activities. Aerobic activity increases the pressure on your lungs and heart resulting in a more efficient pulmonary (heart) and respiratory (lungs) system. Aerobic exercise releases the body's own feel good chemical —endorphins, which boosts your moods, improves your concentration and may reduce the risk of heart disease.

When you engage in aerobic work, your body draws from its available energy sources: stored carbohydrates, fat storage sites and glucose (blood sugar). Carbohydrates are the primary energy source for the first 20 minutes of continuous exercise; it is only <u>after 20 minutes</u> your body switches to its fat reserves for fuel!

Walking is highly recommended for aerobic exercise, its proven ability to remove abdominal fat is legendary. Beginners are encouraged to start with a walking programme. If you are beginning exercise, start with a programme that you are comfortable with.

The Optimum Training Zone

Before discussing aerobic work in detail, I must insist that at all times you adhere carefully to your selected heart rate training zone as it will ensure your safety. To burn calories safely and effectively you must work within <u>your</u> optimum training heart rate zone.

Calculating your MHR (Maximum Heart Rate) may sound daunting but it is an invaluable piece of information for two reasons: 1) It ensures your safety and 2) it enables you to burn fat effectively.

How to Calculate Your Maximum Heart Rate (MHR)

- To calculate your MHR you subtract your age from 220.
- For example if you are 20 years old then your MHR would be 220 - 20 = 200. This figure of 200 is your maximum heart rate (MHR).
- Now you must work out the appropriate % of your MHR for your category.
- If you are a beginner (have not exercised in 6 months) ideally you should work at approximately 60% of your MHR.
- If you are intermediate (have been exercising for over 6months) you can work at 70% to 75% of you MHR.
- If you are advanced you can work at up to 85% of your MHR.

Rate of Perceived Exertion (RPE)

This is a simple yet highly effective tool for monitoring the intensity of your training. The scale is based on your perceived effort which should correlate with your training heart rate. The scale helps you regulate your exertion rate of how hard you perceive it to be, on a scale of one to ten. One is your minimum effort and ten is your maximum. Monitor carefully your effort and adjust accordingly. It allows you understand how your body is reacting to exercise and lets you adjust it accordingly to the activity.

Rest		Gentle		Purposeful		Challenging		Very Tiring	
1	2	3	4	5	6	7	8	9	10
Low activity		Comfortable			Medium		Difficult	Maximum	

The RPE (Rate of Perceived Exertion) Scale

You may monitor and adjust your intensity at any given moment using this technique which is not only accurate but convenient. Choose a number at any given time which best identifies how much effort you are exerting during the workout.

Which level am I?
- An RPE of 4 or less indicates a low intensity workout. Once you move up to 5 you begin to engage in a more strenuous cardiovascular activity.
- An RPE of 5 to 6 indicates a more purposeful activity. You should feel reasonably comfortable and can continue on a conversation without causing undue strain. This level is the normally appropriate for beginners.
- An RPE of 7 to 10 is for advanced seasoned individuals. This indicates a high level of intensity required and will show quick changes to your heart rate and breathing.

To achieve your desired results, you <u>must</u> engage in all activities at the correct intensity. This will ensure your safety while ensuring you work at your optimum heart rate. Identifying your training heart rate is crucial to your success. It allows you to monitor your progress as your body responds to different levels of exertion. This is what is called the overload principle. Your body adapts quickly to any exercise regime, you must constantly strive to increase the repetitions and workload by introducing

variety with different combinations and varying the rest periods. This ensures the muscles are constantly challenged. Why is it important to gauge my exertion? Your heart is a muscle which adapts to different levels of exertion; it becomes stronger as your progress. There are a number of ways to access the intensity at which you are working at.
1. Heart rate—establishing your training heart rate zones.
2. Rate of Perceived exertion

For weight loss, the number of sessions should be between 3 and 4 times per week for a duration of 30 to 45 minutes. If you a beginner, you should strive for 3 times per week for a time span of what you feel comfortable with. If you are a beginner you must get doctors clearance before you start and be monitored by a professional.

To assess your progress, monitor the time of each session. This could range from 15 minutes for a beginner at 60% of their training heart rate to 70 minutes for the advanced. As you gain strength and fitness you will notice results quickly. Always gauge your rate of perceived exertion (RPE). In other words, how you feel during the exercise. How much effort are you exerting? This method helps to regulate your training ensuring you do not over exert yourself. Listen carefully to what your body is telling you. Never ignore its signals! Pay close attention to your suggested RPE and choose a figure from the scale above for an accurate assessment of your work.

The Aerobics Breakthrough

For many years, the aerobic revelation was hailed as the greatest discovery of the fitness world. Aerobic training is often referred to as the foundation stone of any good fitness programme. How does it work? The oxygen you breathe is the fuel required by your body. When you engage in an aerobic activity you increase the rate at which you use oxygen. Your primary objective is to work with your correct "training heart rate" zone as this will ensure you stay within the aerobic zone. If you exert too much pressure you switch to working "an-aerobically" meaning without air. You body will struggle to meet the demands of working without oxygen resulting in exhaustion. Aerobic exercise rekindles the natural instincts of survival; it releases endorphins (happy hormones) into the blood stream creating a general scene of emotional wellbeing helping to fight depression while increasing self-confidence.

There are two types of cardiovascular training.
1. Long steady training: which builds endurance. Long distance walking or running are examples of this type of training.
2. Interval training: which builds stamina, it accelerates your fitness levels by constantly changing the intensity at which you work.

Long steady pace training: fat burner

Allowing your heart rate to work within its designated zones will build long term endurance. It utilises oxygen more efficiently. Long distance runners, swimmers and cyclists use this type of training. This type of training promotes a strong base level of fitness while it guarantees burning off stomach fat. The primary aim is to increase the duration & intensity as you become fitter.

Interval training: Calorie burner

This type of training changes the intensity at which you work, dispelling the myth that only long steady pace training will burn calories. Interval training allows you to work for short bursts of high intensity followed by lower intensity intervals. It enables you to build aerobic strength while increasing your stamina, enabling your respiratory system to function at a higher level. The effect of this type of training is to overload the heart and lungs which stimulates growth and burns calories.

Interval training creates more demands on your heart and lungs. When done under proper supervision, it is the most effective calorie burn. It enables you to burn calories when you are resting due to the increase in your metabolic rate. Interval training creates an "aerobic wave" which will allow your training heart rate to work within its training zone. The aerobic wave is one of the most effective fat burning techniques available.

The Importance of Resistance Training

Scientists have recently discovered the benefits of including resistance training in any weight loss regime. Its virtues can be found in toning, pumping and sculpting your body. Resistance means your muscles have to resist pressure applied to them. So, when you're toning your stomach muscles, you must apply some form of resistance to them in order to work them. This resistance work is crucial for losing weight and re-sculpting your body. The most common forms of resistance training involve using weights, rubber bands or special machines to work the muscles in your body.

Did you know? (Weight training)
Studies have shown that people that have more muscle mass will burn more calories, even at rest. So for long-term weight loss, you will want to incorporate some weight training into your weight loss maintenance plan so that as you increase your calorie intake after a diet, you will then be able to burn them off without any weight gain.

Your muscles are the energy burning, metabolically active part of your body. The better condition they are in, the greater is your ability to burn calories. By applying the "overload principle" you are introducing a new stimulus, as your muscle responds it creates a more efficient calorie burning furnace.

Did you know?
Resistance exercises are the metabolism supercharger!!

Recently, experts in the weight loss and fitness industry suggest that short bursts of cardio are more beneficial than long duration sessions. Some even support the view that cardio training should be avoided completely. From my own experience, I suggest you concentrate on what works! Finding a BALANCE between cardio and resistance training is the most successful method. Latest findings show that maximum fat burning occurs when cardio and resistance training are combined.

In order to successfully lose weight, most people, who have average metabolisms, will have to:
1.   Reduce their calories
2.   Increase their activity

3. Combine cardio with resistance exercises to get the results they want.

For weight maintenance, three cardio sessions per week of 30 to 35 minutes is ideal. For Maximum Fat loss, it is suggested 4 to 6 sessions per week of cardio and resistance training for 35 to 40 minutes working at a moderate intensity. Aerobic and resistance training can be done in the one session. It is important to choose an activity you enjoy. Cycling, using the cross trainer, walking, jogging, swimming or any other continuous activity will yield excellent fat burning results.

Did you know?
In a nutshell, achieving a flat stomach is all about low body fat which is achieved by the burning of excess calories, establishing a healthy eating plan, clean nutrition and most importantly creating a "calorie deficit"

Putting It All Together

The flat stomach programme is possibly the most effective stomach routine ever released. The beauty of this is it can be tailored to suit your lifestyle. You choose if you wish to workout at home or in the gym. If you choose to work at home, you will require only a light set of dumbbells, a Swiss ball and an exercise mat.

Jargon Buster!

Rep = A repetition is one complete movement through an exercise. A simple bicep curl is a great example. You curl your arm up, and then back down. For example if you are told to lift a weight for 12 reps, this means that you repeatedly lift the weight up and down 12 times without stopping.

Set = A set is essentially a group of reps. So if you are asked to do a set of 12 reps then after you have completed 12 reps then you will have completed the set and you should rest for the prescribed period.

Guidelines for Safe and Effective Exercise

Poor technique is responsible for injury, postural defects and a host of medical problems. Incorrect technique can lead to a multitude of injuries. Be sure to follow the tips below for a safe and effective plan.

1. All training MUST be done under professional supervision.
2. All workouts should begin with a 5 minute warm up & stretching and finish with a 5 minute cool down & stretch.
3. Use only the joints and muscles specified for each exercise. Moving your body around too much and using unnecessary movements can cause other muscles to become strained and possibly injured.
4. Breathe correctly. Never hold your breath as it cuts the oxygen supply resulting in blacking out or dizziness. Exhale when exerting pressure, inhale when returning to starting position. Try to synchronize your breathing with the movement.
5. Always cool down using the last 5 minutes to gradually reduce the intensity at which you are working.
6. When performing sit ups, don't swing your body or rush the exercise. Gradually exhale as you move upwards slowly, holding at the top of the contraction for a count of 3 seconds and resist the movement as you slowly return to your starting position. The muscle fibres in your abs are mostly made up of slow twitch fibres, meaning that they actually respond best to slow movements.
7. Work through the full range of motion. The range of motion is the full movement of the exercise. For example, a bicep curl should begin with the arm straight and finish with the fist at the shoulder. If you start with the arm halfway up then you will not work the muscle through its full range of motion.
8. Always strive to progressively increase the number of repetitions.
9. It is important not to overdo exercise. Listen carefully to your body as it will prompt you to respond accordingly. Never ignore its signals.
10. To get the most out of every session, choose activities you enjoy.
11. Keep hydrated – always have a bottle of water to hand.
12. Have a pre-workout light meal (carbohydrates, a banana) 30 minutes before you workout, followed by a post workout (protein) meal within 40 minutes of finishing your workout.

13. Lift weights with the following rhythm: 2 seconds towards you and return it on a count of 4 seconds. Never swing your shoulders.
14. Do sit-ups at the end of each exercise routine, always strive to increase the number of sit-ups you do from the previous day.

The Flat Stomach Workout: Your 30 Day Plan

Let's put all of this information together in the most effective plan possible. What follows is the "30 Days to a Flat Stomach" workout, in which the exercises are grouped together in sets and reps. The primary aim of this plan is to burn body fat while stimulating your metabolic rate through aerobic exercise and targeting your abdominal muscles with most effective stomach exercises available. Warm up with 5 minutes of aerobic exercise, gradually increasing heart rate. Cool down with 5 minutes of decreasing the heart rate followed by full body stretch for all workouts.

Week 1 Day	Duration	Intensity
DAY 1 **Fat-burner**	Warm up 5 mins Walk/run30/40/45min Cool down 5 mins	Beginners: 5/6 Intermediate: 7 Advanced: 8
DAY 2 **Resistance burner**	Warm up 5/7 mins Resistance training Cool down 5 mins	Beginners: 5/6 Intermediate: 7 Advanced: 8
DAY 3 **Calorie-burner**	Warm up 5 mins Aerobic activity 30/40/45 mins Cool down 5 mins	Beginners: 6 Intermediate: 7/8 Advanced: 8
DAY 4	Rest	Rest
DAY 5 **Resistance- burner**	Warm up 5 mins Resistance Training Cool down 5 mins	Beginners: 5/6 Intermediate: 7 Advanced: 8
DAY 6 **Fat-burner**	Warm up 5 mins Walk/run30/35/40 mi Cool down 5 mins	Beginners: 5/6 Intermediate: 7 Advanced: 8
DAY 7 **Resistance-burner**	Warm up 5 mins Resistance Training Cool down 5 mins	Beginners: 5/6 Intermediate: 7 Advanced: 8

Week 2

Day	Duration	Intensity
DAY 1 Fat-burner	Warm up 5 mins Aerobic Activity for 35/45/50min Cool down 5 mins	Beginners: 5/6 Intermediate: 7 Advanced: 8
DAY 2 Resistance burner	Warm up 5/7 mins Resistance training Cool down 5 mins	Beginners: 5/6 Intermediate: 7 Advanced: 8
DAY 3 Calorie-burner	Warm up 5 mins Walk/run 35/45/50min Cool down 5 mins	Beginners: 6 Intermediate: 7/8 Advanced: 8
DAY 4	Rest	Rest
DAY 5 Resistance- burner	Warm up 5 mins Resistance Training Cool down 5 mins	Beginners: 5/6 Intermediate: 7 Advanced: 8
DAY 6 Fat-burner	Warm up 5 mins Walk/run35/45/55 min Cool down 5 mins	Beginners: 5/6 Intermediate: 7 Advanced: 8
DAY 7 Resistance-burner	Warm up 5 mins Resistance Training Cool down 5 mins	Beginners: 5/6 Intermediate: 7 Advanced: 8

Week 3

Day	Duration	Intensity
DAY 1 Fat-burner	Warm up 5 mins Aerobic Activity for 35/45/55min Cool down 5 mins	Beginners: 5/6 Intermediate: 7 Advanced: 8
DAY 2 Resistance burner	Warm up 5/7 mins Resistance training Cool down 5 mins	Beginners: 5/6 Intermediate: 7 Advanced: 8
DAY 3 Calorie-burner	Warm up 5 mins Walk/run Max mins Cool down 5 mins	Beginners: 6 Intermediate: 7/8 Advanced: 8
DAY 4	Rest	Rest
DAY 5 Resistance- burner	Warm up 5 mins Resistance Training Cool down 5 mins	Beginners: 5/6 Intermediate: 7 Advanced: 8
DAY 6 Fat-burner	Warm up 5 mins Walk/run max min Cool down 5 mins	Beginners: 5/6 Intermediate: 7 Advanced: 8
DAY 7 Resistance-burner	Warm up 5 mins Resistance Training Cool down 5 mins	Beginners: 5/6 Intermediate: 7 Advanced: 8

Week 4 Day	Duration	Intensity
DAY 1 Fat-burner	Warm up 5 mins Aerobic Activity for Max min Cool down 5 mins	Beginners: 5/6 Intermediate: 7 Advanced: 8
DAY 2 Resistance burner	Warm up 5/7 mins Resistance training Cool down 5 mins	Beginners: 5/6 Intermediate: 7 Advanced: 8
DAY 3 Calorie-burner	Warm up 5 mins Walk/run max min Cool down 5 mins	Beginners: 6 Intermediate: 7/8 Advanced: 8
DAY 4	Rest	Rest
DAY 5 Resistance- burner	Warm up 5 mins Resistance Training Cool down 5 mins	Beginners: 5/6 Intermediate: 7 Advanced: 8
DAY 6 Fat-burner	Warm up 5 mins Walk/run 45/55/60 min Cool down 5 mins	Beginners: 5/6 Intermediate: 7 Advanced: 8
DAY 7 Resistance-burner	Warm up 5 mins Resistance Training Cool down 5 mins	Beginners: 5/6 Intermediate: 7 Advanced: 8

The above plan gives you a 28 day (4 week) plan. For the final two days of the month go back to week 1 and perform the exercises specified for days 1 and 2. This time, however, you will not be a beginner, so ensure that you perform the exercises at the intermediate or advanced level.

We will now discuss each of the different workout types (fat burner, resistance burner and calorie burner) in some detail, so that you can be confident that you know exactly what to do.

Workout 1: The Fat Burner – Sample Workout			
Exercises	Beginner	Intermediate	Advanced
Walk or Run	30 minutes at 60% of MHR Or 6 on RPE	40 minutes at 70% of MHR Or 7 on RPE	45 minutes at 75% of MHR Or 7.5 RPE

Workout 2: The Resistance Burner – Sample Workout			
Exercises	**Beginner**	**Intermediate**	**Advanced**
Walk/Run	10 minutes at 60% of MHR Or 6 on RPE	10 minutes at 70% of MHR Or 7 on RPE	15 minutes at 75% of MHR Or 7.5 RPE
Press up	1 set of 12 reps	2 sets of 12 reps	3 sets of 12 reps
Dumbbell squat	1 set of 12 reps	2 sets of 12 reps	3 sets of 12 reps
Dumbbell Fly	1 set of 12 reps	2 sets of 12 reps	3 sets of 12 reps
Lunge	1 set of 12 reps	2 sets of 12 reps	3 sets of 12 reps
Triceps dip	1 set of 12 reps	2 sets of 12 reps	3 sets of 12 reps
Bicep curl	1 set of 12 reps	2 sets of 12 reps	3 sets of 12reps
Lateral raise	1 set of 12 reps	2 sets of 12 reps	3 sets of 12 reps

Resistance Training – The Metabolism Booster (MERc)

Resistance training is one of the most productive ways of ensuring lean muscle mass development. The importance of resistance training cannot be over stated. It enhances your overall physical appearance by helping to define those troublesome areas while reclaiming muscle that has gone flabby. It enhances your posture while it strengthens your bone density. It allows you to feel tighter, firmer and gives you a more toned look. If you wish to train in the privacy of your home, get two small dumbbells or improvise with two bottles of water.

As the years pass, muscles which are unused stagnate (this is known as atrophy). Resistance training restores the muscle and promotes the essential fat burning which is necessary for weight loss. Once you pass the age of thirty, you begin to lose muscle which signals a slower rate of calorie burning which explains why it is easy to put on weight as you get older. As the muscles weaken, it opens the door to an array of health issues, postural problems, lower back injuries, bone density deterioration as well as having a soft, flabby figure which also has physiological ramifications.

During resistance training, the muscle tissue is broken down and is rebuilt with aid of protein; this process takes up to 48 hours. That is why it is strongly advised to take protein within 40 minutes of finishing a workout. This is called the "Golden window". Replacing soft muscle tissue with a lean metabolically active muscle tissue not only gives you a leaner more defined look but also has many positive physical and psychological benefits.

Did you know?
Women find it extremely difficult to add muscle due to the presence of oestrogen in their bodies. This means that it is practically impossible for women to obtain a "muscle man" look from doing resistance training. This is a concern of many women but you can rest assured that this will not happen. If you see a woman with this look then it is most likely that she has used illegal steroids in order to obtain this body shape.

Lunge

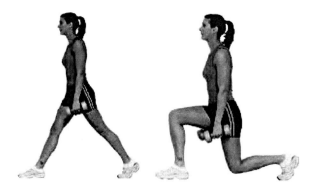

Hold two light dumbbells in each hand alongside your body. Keep your arms straight. Place feet shoulder width apart, step forward with the right leg and allow the left heel to rise off the ground. Keep your back straight and engage your core muscles by contracting your stomach muscles. Now move in a downward motion until your right hamstring (muscle at the back of your tight) is parallel to the ground. From this position move upwards and down until you have completed the required number of repetitions. Once completed, repeat the same format on your left leg.

Dumbbell Military press

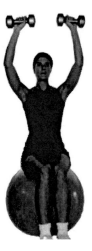

Sit on a bench or a chair with a dumbbell in each hand. Keeping your back straight with your feet shoulder width apart, raise the dumbbells to shoulder level. Press dumbbells in an upward motion until the dumbbells meet at the top of the movement. Do not lock your elbows at the top of the movement. Slowly return the dumbbells until to shoulder level and repeat for the required number of repetitions. Engage your core muscles by tensing your stomach muscles during the exercise.

Bicep curl

Sit on a bench or chair, place your feet together, back straight while holding a dumbbell in each hand facing away from you. Image your elbow is glued onto the side of your stomach and cannot move. Place the dumbbells in your hands with your palms facing away from you. Rotate both dumbbells in an upward motion without moving your elbow until your palm is parallel to your shoulder and gently return to the starting position. Repeat the suggested number of sets and repetitions.

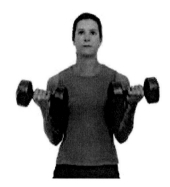

Dumbbell press

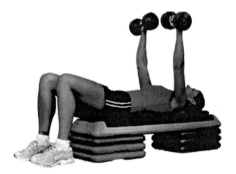

This exercise will help to reshape your chest area and, if you are a lady will do wonders for your bust; this is done by strengthening your pectoral muscles or "pecs" as they are commonly known. Lie on a flat bench holding both dumbbells in each hand. Place the dumbbells in line with your nipples. Your palms should be facing away from you. Now, push the dumbbells away from you body until your arms are almost straight. Avoid locking the elbows at the end of the pressing/pushing movement. Lower the dumbbells on a count of 4 seconds and do the suggested number of repetitions.

Triceps dip

This exercise will help to define and tone your triceps. The triceps muscle is located at the back of your arms and is a well know fat deposit site. Place both hands behind you on a chair or bench. Your hands should be supporting your weight. Gently lower your bottom towards the ground. Allow for a full or partial range of movement (whatever you feel comfortable with). Lower yourself on a count of 4 seconds finishing with your upper arms parallel with the floor. Slowly return to the starting position, doing the required number of repetitions.

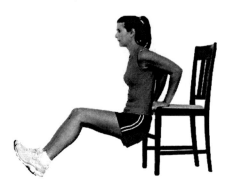

All the above exercises should be done to the following set/rep count:

Resistance Burner – Workout Planner			
Week	**Beginner**	**Intermediate**	**Advanced**
Week 1	1 set of 12 reps	2 sets of 12 reps	3 sets of 12 reps
Week 2	2 set of 12 reps	3 sets of 12 reps	4 sets of 12 reps
Week 3	2 sets of 15 reps	3 sets of 15 reps	4 sets of 15 reps
Week 4	2 sets of 20 reps	3 sets of 20 reps	4 sets of 20 reps

Summary of the Benefits of Weight Training

- It re-shapes your body
- It develops metabolically active muscle (Meaning it burns more calories than fat).
- You may burn calories for a further 24 hours after you exercise.

- It increases your bone density.
- It is strongly recommended as prevention to osteo-porosis.
- It burns away fat deposit sites.
- It removes cellulite
- It may firm stubborn residual body fat.
- It supports anti aging.

10

Get Bikini Ready in Just 21 Days!

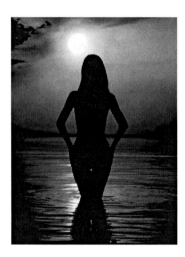

The 21 Day Blitz!

The first signs of summer are usually the trigger for most people to shape up and shift the extra pounds which have become firmly lodged around the mid rift over the winter months. As the layers of clothing which were needed for those cold months are now abandoned, the thoughts of having to be seen in a swimsuit as the holidays approach can be daunting. It can often be a rash decision which is motivated the fear of looking fat on the beach. So how can you get into shape without having to take drastic measures such as surgery or going on a starvation diet for weeks? Perhaps you are one of the many who dread the prospect of spending hours cooked up in a sweaty gym? Or maybe feel intimidated by the bouncing beauties that seem to spend every waking moment exercising in the gym!

Shaping up does not have to entail starving yourself or temporarily relocating to the gym. This twenty one day eating plan will help whittle down your waistline by removing toxins from your daily diet and replacing them with healthy natural alternatives.

Size Really Does Matter

The suggested portion size of protein per meal is approximately the size of your palm and the suggested guideline for your carbohydrate intake is twice the area between your knuckles when your fist is closed.

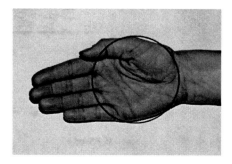

Suggested Portion Size for Protein: The size of your palm

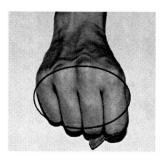

The Suggested Portion Size for Carbohydrates is twice the size of the area between your knuckles when you make a fist.

The following guidelines give the main points of this eating plan:
- You should eat carbohydrates AND proteins together.
- Apply the 90/10 rule. Be good for 90% of the time which allows you to indulge for 10% of the time.
- Choose organic foods as they contain fewer toxins and have more health boosting minerals and vitamins.
- Avoid sugar cravings by making sure to eat every two hours. Sugar cravings come from a lack of protein in your eating plan. Try having non salted nuts when you feel hungry. They are a wonderful source of protein and fill you up quickly.

- Consume green vegetables every day, in a blender or in their natural form.
- Remember your five a day and consume five pieces of fruit daily.

The 21 Day Bikini Eating Plan

Day One

Breakfast	Muesli and two pieces of fruit
11 am	Banana
Lunch	One grilled fish, rocket leaves, red peppers and chopped onions
4 pm	Apple
Dinner	100g of red meat, steamed green vegetables and a cup of brown rice
8.30 pm	Organic yogurt with a handful of non salted mixed nuts

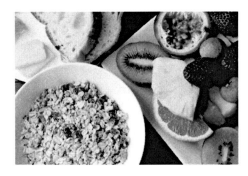

Day Two

Breakfast	Oatmeal with a spoonful of natural honey
11 am	Apple
Lunch	Two slices of white meat, rocket leaves, red peppers and cucumber
4 pm	Pear
Dinner	100g of steamed or grilled fish, steamed green beans and a baked potato
8.30 pm	Organic yogurt with two pieces of fruit mixed in

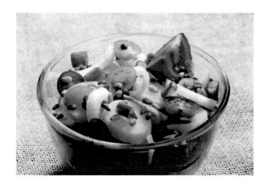

Day Three

Breakfast	Omelette with spinach and a cup of green tea
11 am	Cup full of non salted nuts
Lunch	Bowl of minestrone soup and one slice of wholemeal bread
4 pm	Pear
Dinner	100g of grilled chicken with steamed green beans and a cupful of wild rice.
8.30 pm	Organic yogurt

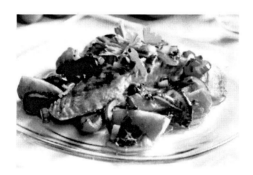

Day Four

Breakfast	Oatmeal with a spoonful of natural honey
11 am	Banana
Lunch	Grilled sea bass, tomatoes and green vegetables
4 pm	Peach
Dinner	Feta cheese with olives, green beans and a cupful of wild rice
8.30 pm	Avocado

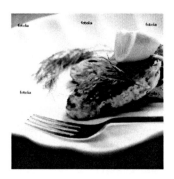

Day Five

Breakfast	Scrambled eggs with mushrooms
11 am	Slice of melon
Lunch	Tuna mixed with fresh green salad
4 pm	Cup full of Brazilian nuts
Dinner	Breast of chicken, broccoli and one baked potato
8.30 pm	Two oatmeal biscuits

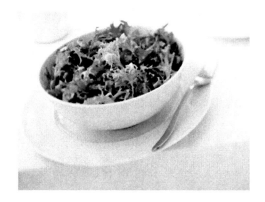

Day Six

Breakfast	Mixed fruit salad with seeds and nuts mixed in
11 am	Apple
Lunch	Homemade beef burger with grilled mushrooms and onions served with a side salad
4 pm	Slice of melon
Dinner	Grilled mackerel or salmon with a stir fry of mixed seasoned vegetables
8.30 pm	Avocado

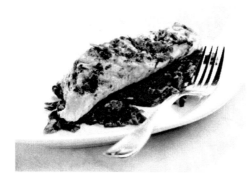

Day Seven

Breakfast	Poached egg with one slice of wholemeal bread
11 am	Banana
Lunch	Pan fried prawns with mixed salad
4 pm	Cupful of non salted nuts
Dinner	Grilled fillet of salmon with a cupful of humus and a portion of green vegetables
8.30 pm	Two rice cakes

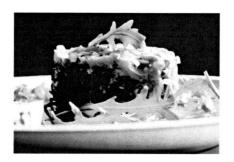

Day Eight

Breakfast	Oatmeal with a spoonful of natural honey
11 am	Pear
Lunch	Roast chicken with green bean salad with a squeeze of lemon
4 pm	Cupful of non salted nuts
Dinner	Skewers filled with steak or sole and cherry tomatoes
8.30 pm	Avocado

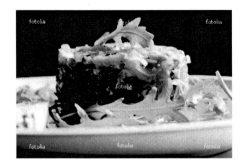

Day Nine

Breakfast	Spinach omelette
11 am	Slice of water melon
Lunch	Bowl of vegetable soup with two slices of wholemeal bread
4 pm	Cupful of non salted nuts
Dinner	100g of turkey, one baked potato and a selection of green chopped vegetables
8.30 pm	Two rice cakes

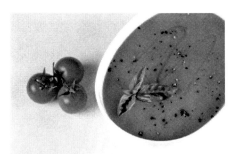

Day Ten

Breakfast	Mixed fruit salad with nuts mixed in
11 am	Organic yogurt with seeds mixed in
Lunch	Grilled tuna steak, a cupful of hummus and side salad
4 pm	Cupful of mixed non salted nuts
Dinner	100g of goat's cheese, finely chopped tomatoes and red onions.
8.30 pm	Two oatmeal biscuits

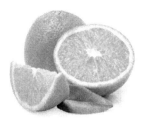

Day Eleven

Breakfast	Scrambled eggs with tomato and mushrooms
11 am	Two rice cakes
Lunch	Grilled chicken breast with a cupful of wild rice and a side salad
4 pm	Apple
Dinner	100g of beef with sautéed vegetables and a cupful or hummus or one baked potato
8.30 pm	Organic yogurt with banana mixed through

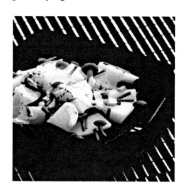

Day Twelve

Breakfast	Poached eggs on a slice of wholemeal bread
11 am	Pear
Lunch	Leek and Potato soup with two pieces of Rye crackers
4 pm	Red apple
Dinner	Grilled fillet of salmon with cucumbers, one tomato and grapes
8.30 pm	Two oatmeal biscuits

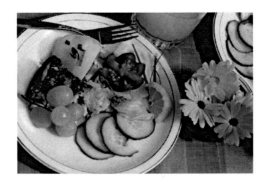

Day Thirteen

Breakfast	Organic oatmeal with linseed mixed through
11 am	Slice of water melon
Lunch	Grilled sea trout with steamed courgettes or sushi rolls
4 pm	Two bananas
Dinner	Roast chicken with a cupful of hummus and a portion of finely chopped vegetables
8.30 pm	Organic yogurt with cashew nuts.

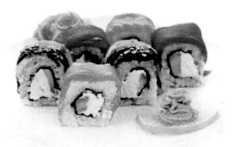

Day Fourteen

Breakfast	Mixed fruit salad with seeds and nuts
11 am	Cupful of non salted nuts
Lunch	Grilled mackerel with a portion of finely chopped onions and a cupful of hummus or rice
4 pm	Two apples
Dinner	100g of rump steak, pan-fried mushrooms and onions with a cupful of mashed potato
8.30 pm	Two oatcakes

Days Fifteen to Twenty One

On these days you may pick your favourite seven menus from those listed above and use them. Make sure you pick seven different menus though! Do not just pick one or two days and repeat them. Variety is important in this eating plan.

Things You Must do Each Day

- Include as many low glycaemic (low GI) foods as possible.
- 70% of your eating plan should be made up of natural foods
- Allow one cup of coffee per day.
- Limit the units of alcohol to 7 per week.
- Drink at least two full glasses of water with each meal.
- Graze: eat every two to two and a half hours.
- Eliminate sugary drinks such as sodas and fizzy drinks.
- Consume five pieces of fruit daily.
- Consume green vegetables daily.
- Take one cup of green tea daily
- Try eating non salted nuts when hungry
- Consume protein as the last meal of the day.
- Combine protein with carbohydrates.
- Eliminate junk and fast foods from you eating plan.
- Become sugar & salt free
- Remove processed and convenience food from your eating plan.
- Eat avocado pears

The 21 Day Bikini Workout (No Gym Required!)

The primary aim is to look slim and toned in your swimsuit, so the main focus is to lose excess body fat. Twenty one days is not long so you must focus. This programme includes high intensity aerobic and resistance training, which includes switching from low intensity to high intensity work. It also promotes higher levels of fitness while increasing your metabolic rate (the rate at which you burn calories). Once the body fat begins to melt away, the resistance training will tone up your chosen areas. Women tend pile on extra pounds around the mid-riff. This programme targets stomach fat and creates a lean and toned stomach. Once this has been achieved, it accentuates the upper body.

Equipment Needed

Any exercise aimed at toning your body needs something to provide resistance for your muscles to work against. Select a set of dumbbells ranging from 1lb-5lb/0.5-2kg.

Timing and Repetitions

12 reps of each exercise is the suggested number of repetitions. Allow for a 5 minute warm up and 5 minute cool down with each session. Walking up and down your stairs or marching on the spot is ideal solution. Stretch before and after you have exercised.

How to Workout

Do three days straight followed by one day rest. Do cardiovascular one day followed by a resistance the next; follow the three day on one day off rule for the entire 21 days of the programme. Remember to always check with your doctor or GP before you commence a new exercise programme.

The tables below show how you should exercise. For the cardiovascular exercise (aerobic exercise) you should choose one of the activities listed and do that activity for the length of time listed and the RPE (rate of perceived exertion) shown. The RPE scale is shown again below for your convenience.

Rest		Gentle		Purposeful		Challenging		Very Tiring	
1	2	3	4	5	6	7	8	9	10
Low activity		Comfortable			Medium		Difficult	Maximum	

The RPE (Rate of Perceived Exertion) Scale

Cardiovascular Workout			
Exercise	Beginner	Intermediate	Advanced
Walking or Cycling or Swimming or Jogging	As long as possible RPE = 5	Minimum of 30 mins RPE = 6-7	Minimum of 45 mins RPE = 7-8

108

Resistance Workout						
Exercise	Beginners 2 Sets	RPE	Intermediate 4 Sets	RPE	Advanced 4 Sets	RPE
Press up	12 reps	5	10 reps	7	12 reps	7
	Max reps	6	8 reps	8	10 reps	8
			Max reps	8	Max reps	9
			Max reps	8	Max reps	9
Bridge	12 reps	5	10 reps	7	12 reps	7
	Max reps	6	8 reps	8	10 reps	8
			Max reps	8	Max reps	9
			Max reps	8	Max reps	9
Triceps dip	12 reps	5	10 reps	7	12 reps	7
	Max reps	6	8 reps	8	10 reps	8
			Max reps	8	Max reps	9
			Max reps	8	Max reps	9
Squat	12 reps	5	10 reps	7	12 reps	7
	Max reps	6	8 reps	8	10 reps	8
			Max reps	8	Max reps	9
			Max reps	8	Max reps	9
Lunge	12 reps	5	10 reps	7	12 reps	7
	Max reps	6	8 reps	8	10 reps	8
			Max reps	8	Max reps	9
			Max reps	8	Max reps	9
Sit Up	12 reps	5	10 reps	7	12 reps	7
	Max reps	6	8 reps	8	10 reps	8
			Max reps	8	Max reps	9
			Max reps	8	Max reps	9

For the resistance workout you should complete the number of sets and repetitions shown in the table above. "Max reps" means you should do as many of the exercise as possible until your muscles are so tired that you cannot complete any more. You should rest for 30 seconds in between sets. I will now describe how to do each resistance exercise in detail.

Exercise 1 - Press-ups

Kneel on a mat and place both hands a little wider than your shoulders, contract your abdominal muscles. Bend your elbows and touch your chin off the mat, exhaling as you push yourself back up to your starting position. Repeat for the required number of reps.

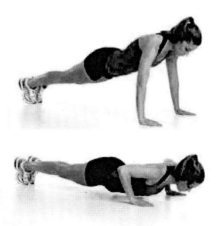

Exercise 2 – The Plank

Lie face down on the mat, position yourself so that your toes are on the ground and your elbows are directly under your shoulders. Lift yourself up, keeping a straight line from your ankles, so your body is being supported by your toes and your elbows. Contract your abdominal muscles.

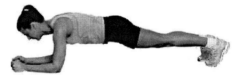

Exercise 3- Triceps dips

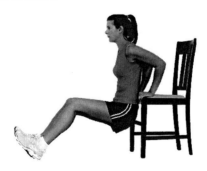

Use a chair or a small table and ensure it is supported against a wall. Place your feet hip width apart, keep your back straight. Place both hands behind you on the chair and slowly lower yourself down until your arms are bent at 90 degrees, then push yourself back up until your arms are straight, but do not lock out your arms at the end of the motion. You should feel the backs of your arms (triceps muscles) being worked Repeat as required.

Exercise 4- Squat

Stand upright with your feet hip-width apart and your knees slightly bent. Keep your back straight while placing your hands on your hips; bend your knees to 90 degrees allowing your body to lean forward gently until it is at right angles to your thighs while keeping your heels on the floor. Exhale as you exert pressure. Repeat as required. You can use a chair, as shown below, as a guide: when your bottom touches the chair then your knees will be at 90 degrees. Don't sit down in this case – just touch the chair with your bottom and then move straight up again.

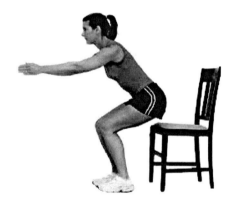

Exercise 5 - Lunge

Standing upright, place one foot forward about one metre ahead of your back leg, keep your hip facing outwards and place your hands on your hips or you can hold a set of dumbbells. Keep your body upright. Now bend your knees to bring your forward knee directly over your front foot. Hold for a count of 4 seconds and return to your starting position. After you have done the suggested numbers of repetitions do the same on the other leg.

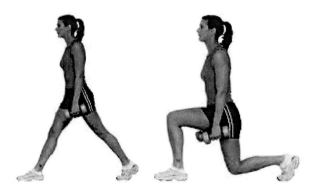

Exercise 6 - Sit ups

Lie on a mat facing the ceiling. Slightly bend your knees with your feet flat on the floor with your hands over your earlobes. Slowly raise your chest towards your knees. At the top of the contraction hold for a count of 4 seconds and slowly return to your starting position. This is usually quite a small range of movement. When returning to the starting position, do not allow your shoulders to touch the ground.

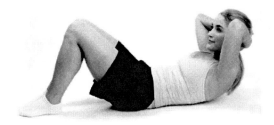

11

How do the Super Models do it?

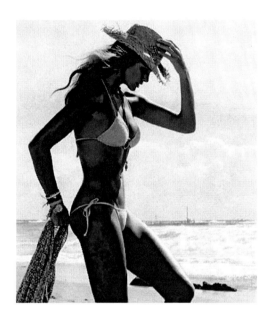

The Secret Revealed

It can't be easy being a supermodel these days, but how do they manage to look so good? Have they been gifted with some supernatural genes? Supermodel turned entrepreneur Elle Macpherson knows only too well the hidden truth of looking great. She has become the envy of most of most middle aged women as she approaches her 50th birthday. Elle recently revealed that it takes time and effort to keep her enviable figure in great shape. "I don't run eight miles a day like I used to. I eat a lot of organic food and drink lots of water, and I take time for meditation to set up my day." As well as working out, she practices Pilates, yoga and sports such as water-skiing, hiking, surfing and paddle boarding. The pursuit of looking good can take hours out of her day - a luxury that most of us can rarely afford. Some celebrities claim that they are genetically predisposed with high metabolisms enabling them to eat vast amounts of food and forgo the gym. If truth be told, this is rarely the case. Elle has been bestowed with wonderful body structure but it is an everyday struggle to maintain peak condition. When recently asked by a journalist how she maintains her stunning figure she replied "I live by the rule: what you eat you crave". Wise words!

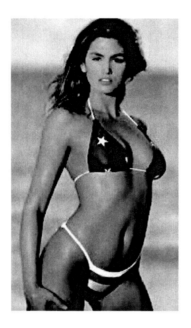

Cindy Crawford is also quick to echo the sentiments of her former colleague. She admits to be being good 80% of the time and allowing herself to indulge the other 20%. "We all know when we are blowing it, but as long as you don't do it all of the time it is generally ok". She is also militant about her daily eating regime. Breakfast is oatmeal and berries and lunch is usually white meat and salad. It is important to realise that men and women's metabolism slows down once they pass the mid thirties and they begin to lose muscle mass. This invariability means that staying in peak condition becomes more challenging.

Adriana Lima is one of the world's top models; she recently shared her secrets for keeping in top shape. Her average daily diet consisted of:

Breakfast   Egg whites, oatmeal and raisins or muesli with

	plain yogurt and honey, along with milk
Lunch	A portion of meat (fish, chicken or red meat) with veggies
Snacks	Raw veggies such as cucumbers and carrots. She does indulge her sweet tooth with chocolate too! She also has a daily spoonful of raw honey explaining "it helps your immune system."
Dinner	Small salad. She says she sleeps better at night when she eats light later in the day.

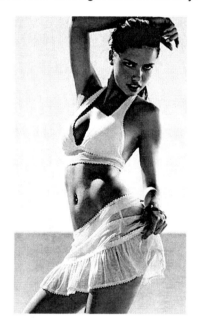

Adriana follows the "Portion Control Diet" which basically means she is allowed to eat everything she wants, but only in small bites if it is unhealthy or high in fat. That doesn't mean she eats junk food all day; but she can have a piece of fat food or even a high calorie food as long as it is a small portion size. This portion control diet has turned her body into a fat burning machine.

Adriana also exercises to stay in shape. She does Brazilian martial arts combining dance, music aerobics and choreographed play fighting, and other cardio workouts. With her portion control and regular exercise routine, Adriana has turned her body into an automatic fat burning machine. Changing your body so that it automatically burns fat is the best thing you can do for your body. In almost everything I read about Adriana Lima there were two things she always mentioned when talking about dieting or healthy living: 1. Drink lots of water and 2. Get plenty of sleep.

The theory that a high metabolism is the answer for their remarkable shape is redundant. They all share one common denominator they work really hard at it. An envious figure requires time, discipline and effort. There are no easy solutions.

12

Emotional Eating – The Solution

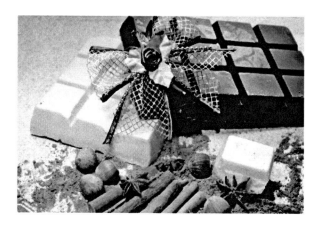

Banish Emotional Eating Forever

Latest research suggests that up to 75% of overeating is caused by emotions. To key is to understand why you eat when you feel emotionally challenged. Your appetite is governed by biochemical transmitters which send signals to brain when you are hungry or thirsty. These signals are often ignored when you feel low or anxious and eating becomes a comfort mechanism to mask some unpleasant situation. For many of us we have become conditioned to believe food is a way rewarding ourselves for a task successfully completed. As we grow older, food often becomes a substitute for something lacking in our lives. Indulging in empty calories temporarily fills a void but at what cost?

The consumption of large quantities of comfort food, usually junk will cause a major upset to your blood sugars, weight and emotional wellbeing. Many people associate pleasure with food, resulting in turning to food to console themselves when they feel upset. It is likely that an underlying physiological issue needs to be addressed. By identifying your trigger situations, you can replace emotional eating with a positive technique, eliminating weight gain and fluctuating blood sugars from the equation. The daily pressures of life take their toll. Balancing family commitments with a career, meeting deadlines etc can you leave you emotionally drained? There will be times when you might be tempted to throw in the towel and return to your comfort zone. At times like this the best remedy is <u>rest</u> and <u>company</u>. Never allow yourself to be on your own.

Real hunger is a natural response of your brain signalling a message from your stomach to take in nourishing foods which will replenish its fuel reserves. Learn to recognise the signs of real hunger:

- Real hunger builds gradually
- Real hunger is satisfied with healthy, nutritious foods
- With real hunger, you are satisfied after you eat and feel full.

Emotional hunger is a hunger you feel when there is a void in your life or you are feeling anxious or depressed. The need to fill that void is often a response to deeper unresolved issues. After you have indulged, you will feel guilty. Learn to recognise the signs of emotional hunger:

- Emotional hunger comes on suddenly
- Emotional hunger tends to come in the form of cravings for a specific food - many times this will be fatty, salty or sugary
- Emotional eating is always followed by feeling of guilt and self-loathing.

The Domino Effect

Emotional eating sets off a chain of negative events. Firstly it is usually done at night, with junk food being the main culprit sending your blood sugars soaring followed by a sudden drop, leaving you feeling bloated and rotten. Your energy is depleted, now you feel miserable, emotional and tired. This is accompanied by another sugar craving, fuelling the cycle. Your willpower has evaporated, you feel depressed, and so you comfort yourself by eating more. You may feel you have blown it so what does it matter if you indulge again? The cycle takes on a life of its own. As it progresses, another more important factor enters the equation. You feel guilty. At this point there are two directions you can go:

1. You firmly resolve to get back on track and you do.
2. You give up, making you feel utterly miserable. Your self esteem hits rock bottom.

Everything goes back to your self esteem, whatever you can do to build your self esteem you must pursue, whatever diminishes your self esteem you should avoid. Proper nutrition and exercise are your two best assets for building your self confidence. I have experienced the never ending cycle of emotional eating, the junk quickly followed by the resolution, it was only when I identified my trigger points that I could pre-empt another episode. Until you break this cycle, you remain chained to the misery of emotional eating both physically and physiologically. The causes of the condition have not yet been identified; there are a number of factors which you may recognise. Identify the appropriate ones for you.

The main emotional eating triggers are:
- Feeling depressed.
- Feeling overwhelmed.
- Unconsciously sabotaging your efforts to change
- Feeling hurt or betrayed
- Feeling tired or rundown
- Low self esteem
- Boredom
- A dependency on highly refined sugary foods
- Chemically altered foods
- Convenience foods
- Fast food
- Microwaving
- Lack of sunlight
- Excessive working hours
- Stress
- Dehydration
- Toxic eating habits

Prioritise three causes from above list. Identifying your eating triggers is the first step; this alone is not enough to alter your eating habits. Once you have identified the emotional thought pattern you must break the cycle.

Substituting an alternative positive habit is the second step. Now replace eating with some form of positive activity that you really enjoy, such as:

- Reading
- Going for a walk
- Relaxing scented bath
- Cinema
- Meeting with friends
- Playing a game of Golf

So for example,
1. Feeling depressed --replace eating with a scented bath.
2. Feeling bored --replace this with meeting a friend.
3. Feeling Stressed --replace eating with a massage.

Pre-empt negative eating with a positive response. This in turn releases a positive chain of events. Firstly you feel great because you are eating properly; physiologically you will feel stronger for not having given in to the dreaded temptation and thirdly, your self-esteem will be enhanced.

Did you know?
Emotional eating always leaves you feeling rotten.

If you are not getting the full range of minerals or vitamins daily, you can take a multivitamin which will address this. Jogging or power walking reduces stress or tension. Pilates or a massage will assist in the removal of stress. Establishing proper sleeping patterns will improve your moods and your wellbeing. The biggest factor which contributes to emotional eating are low self esteem, depression, loneliness and anxiety. It may be a combination of two or more of the above. By eating foods which have being chemically altered, reinforces the cycle. Keep yourself hydrated at all times, if you feel you need water it is too late as you are already dehydrated. Water acts as a coolant and a cleansing agent to your cells. The single most important ingredient for breaking the emotional eating cycle is to avoid fast food and junk, it is imperative. Modern day living is full of challenges, by consuming fresh organic food and exercising you cannot feel bad, you are respecting yourself by filling up with healthy food.

Research suggests that the most powerful technique for breaking negative habits is visualisation, to see yourself breaking this addiction, seeing that image of how you will look, knowing you are going to achieve it. See yourself exactly how you want to look, get an image and look at it daily, then work to make it happen. You will achieve your heart's desire.

Mind-Body Link

Everything starts in your mind; your emotions dictate the quality of your life. You must nourish your mind as well as your body. Paradoxically it is your physical wellbeing which influences your mental wellness. By eating correctly, getting adequate rest, and exercising you feel good about yourself; your self-esteem improves which in turn allows you to cope better with life's challenges. By addressing your physical needs, you are enhancing your mental wellness, which responds by supporting your physical health. They are inseparable; one is feeding off the other. Never be afraid to take time out and seek help if you are not feeling well.

11 Ways to Improve Your Mood

Changing your moods is not difficult if you follow the following guidelines. Implementing small daily lifestyle changes can have a profound impact on your moods and wellbeing. A number of factors will influence your moods on any given day, including what you have eaten and what time you have eaten it at. Dehydration and sleep deprivation are two of the most common symptoms for feeling low.

The implementation of these simple steps will have a profound impact on your moods and wellbeing. When you feel low, your moods seep into every area of your life. There is a constant battle to stay motivated.

1. Wheat intolerance: Wheat is one of the corner stone's of our diet and also one of the hardest things to try and avoid. Often it can be found in foods that we would least expect. Most types of bread are wheat based; this includes "rye" and "corn" loaves which often contain some wheat. As a rule try to avoid wheat.

2. Sunlight & Vitamin D: vitamin D helps the body to absorb calcium and phosphate, which are both essential for bone growth and repair. Research from Columbia University and the Harvard Medical School suggest that vitamin D in combination with parathyroid hormone may actually increase bone density, which would enable older people to fight against osteoporosis. Sunlight is an excellent source of vitamin D.

3. Moods and foods: Latest research has highlighted the link between our moods and the foods we chose. By carefully selecting foods rich in natural vitamins and minerals have many mood enhancing agents. Gorging on processed foods will destabilise your blood sugars creating sugar spikes and dips which in turn will guarantee you feeling miserable.

4. Stable blood sugars: In order for you to function at your optimal levels, you must stabilise your blood sugars. This is achieved by eating every two hours. If you allow your body to go without foods for long periods of time it only destabilises your blood sugars resulting in sugar craving.

5. Oily fish: Try to make oily fish a large part of your weekly eating plan. They provide a rich source of minerals, nutrients and essential fats; they have countless health benefits and provide fatty acids which are the building blocks of the brain. These acids are only found in any significant amounts   in oily fish and fish oils.

6. Feeling tired?: Often when we feel tired or run down we choose sugar and coffee as artificial stimulants to perk us up. The truth is you become hyperactive due to these artificial stimulants resulting in finding it impossible to switch off. This begins the cycle of taking more artificial stimulants to help you relax, taking more you to perk you up. It becomes endless.

7. Sleep: In order to improve your moods, you must get adequate sleep. Remember the last time you felt drained? Your world can become a very dark and hostile place. Sleep is one of the most beneficial ways to improve your moods.

8. Fresh Air: Did you know that your body is made up of trillions of cells? Each of those tiny cells needs a constant supply of oxygen in order to live. We can only live for a few minutes without air. Fresh air is an instant energiser while improving your mood.

9. Exercise: When you exercise you automatically release endorphins—the body own feel good chemicals. Remember

the last time you exercised? You cannot help but feel great after it.

10. Oatmeal in the morning: Oatmeal is low glycaemic which means it is gently released into the blood streams. It also has the benefit of keeping you feeling full up to lunchtime.

11. Combine Protein and carbohydrates: this gives a full feeling and also an immediate energy boost. It reduces the chances of snacking and also stabilises your blood sugars.

13

Putting it All Together

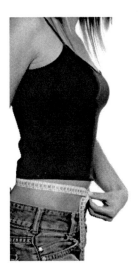

When the Going Gets Tough

To achieve lasting success, you must be prepared to keep highly motivated. Persistence is possibly the most common thread running through the lives of people who have achieved extraordinary achievements. There may be moments of doubt, frustration and anger as you pursue your goal. At times you may feel the universe is plotting against you! It may be challenging but nothing tastes as good as knowing you are on the road to success. These are just pitfalls and you can learn to handle these as merely a natural part of your progression. Once you mastered these obstacles, it instils a scene of pride as you realise your full potential.

The Magic Light Switch

Locked away inside your brain is a magic light switch. When it is the ON position it is empowering you with positive responses: it is fuelling your imagination with positive images of how you will look and how you will feel when you achieve your goal. It is absolutely critical to keep this imaginary light switch in the ON position. Once this light switch is in the ON position, you are motivated, positive and steadily moving in the right direction. It is only a matter of time before your goal becomes your reality.

If that light switch goes to the OFF position, it is only a matter of time before you give up. You must do anything that is required to support the ON position, even if it means having a cheat day or indulging in whatever is your vice! If you feel deprived, this is warning signal to modify your behaviour immediately to allow whatever it is you want in moderation. As a rule: have the least amount you will get away with.

Top Tips for Staying Positive

- Seeking out good information or books on proper nutrition and exercise will enhance your mental state.
- Find role models and ask for their advice or research their methods on the internet or through books/magazines.
- Find a training buddy who will help to motivate you. Latest research shows that you are more likely to stick with a programme if you have company.
- Find an exercise/diet plan that can be customised to you and which you enjoy.
- Seek out a variety of different foods and exercises which will keep you stimulated.
- Reward yourself daily for consistently meeting your targets
- Mentally visualize the end result of your efforts.

Play tricks with your mind: the single most important goal is to keep the positivity switched on. Play tricks and reward yourself daily for completing your tasks. You must also keep your routine interesting, once you are familiar with it, change it. Never allow yourself to stagnate. Repeat positive affirmations daily. Understanding the complexity of the human mind is your key to unlocking the door to success. There are positive states of mind which empower you like love, respect, joy, inner harmony and peace. These positive states of mind allow you access to the great hidden untapped powers of your subconscious mind. Likewise, negativity is a like festering cancer spreading throughout your body. It can immobilise your enthusiasm, and destroy your dreams leaving you angry, frustrated and confused. Persistence is the key!

Take a leaf out of the book of some of the world's leading athletes and visualize the end result. Imagine the way you will look when you have that elusive toned flat stomach. Imagine the pride you will feel. Imagine the clothes you can wear without feeling embarrassed. Now harness that energy into achieving it.

3 Simple Lifestyle Secrets for an Even Healthier You

Reshaping your stomach is more than just a function of your eating and exercising plan. It is important to consider lifestyle changes which will ensure lasting success. If you find it very challenging to remove that last few remaining pounds from around your mid-section, it could be lifestyle choices which are responsible.

Secret 1: Sleep Secrets

Most people have difficulty in waking up in the morning. Recent studies have found that sleep is one of the important components for your overall wellness. If your sleep patterns are disturbed on a regular basis, it disrupts your entire lifestyle. It may lead to anxiety, feelings of being overwhelmed or just being grumpy. Lack of sleep triggers an eating response; studies have found someone who is not getting adequate sleep requires up to 30% more Carbohydrates than a person who is getting their nightly quota.

Lack of sleep may be responsible for slowing down your metabolism, which prevents your body from using glucose which is stored ready for use. Also, a lack of sleep can affect your serotonin level which in turn controls your moods. Broken sleep patterns can leave you feeling deflated, groggy and lifeless. Sleep deprivation impedes the efficiency at which your growth hormones functions. During rest, your body repairs injuries and helps rebalance your energy. It supports the removal of toxins from your system and helps to dissipate stress.

Top Tips for Enhancing Your Sleep Patterns

- Your sleep patterns are controlled by an internal clock. Routine is the key to establishing lasting sleep patterns. If this routine is disturbed, it may cause difficulties in establishing the routine again. One night of disrupted sleep will not cause a difficulty but try to adhere to the same going to bed time each day where possible.
- Limit caffeine: the more dependent you are on artificial stimuli the harder it will be to wake up. Limit yourself to one cup of coffee per day, and try switching from normal tea to herbal tea.
- Ensuring your bedroom is dark and well ventilated will improve the quality of your sleep.
- How do you know if you are getting enough sleep? If you need an alarm clock to wake up then unfortunately you are not getting enough sleep! If you get enough sleep you should wake naturally at the time you wish to get up.
- You will naturally emerge from sleep when your body feels adequately rested.
- Try to use the last 2 hours before you go to sleep as a winding down process. Read a book, take a relaxing bath and don't take phone calls late at night where possible.
- Drink 3 cups of camomile tea daily, as it has a calming effect.

Secret 2: Stay Positive

When you are feeling low, your body overproduces a hormone called cortisol. In the presence of cortisol the fat cells in your abdominal area respond by increasing in size. Research shows that people who are heavy caffeine users or under undue stress create a "fight or flight" response. Recent studies have found that people who are under constant stress or have gone through a traumatic experience have excess weight around their mid-sections due to their circumstances. The University of California in San Francisco put 59 pre-menopausal women through a stress test. They discovered that women with a higher percentage of abdominal fat preformed poorer by secreting more cortisol than those who had a lower abdominal body fat. What this study highlights is the greater stress levels you experience contribute to a higher fat distribution around the midsection. Cortisol is the hormonal agent responsible for this.

If you are experiencing a stress related event, you should incorporate stress management into your daily routine.

Prioritise: If, like most people, you are overcommitted to your career, family responsibilities or housekeeping errands you need to step back and prioritise your day, ensuring you get balance and clarity back into your life. Incorporate rest and relaxation into every day as it will rejuvenate you.

Stay focused: What are your key areas to rebalance your life? At times when there are so many demands made on you it can leave you overwhelmed, disillusioned and exhausted. The world can lose it magic as you are subjected to one crisis after another. The next time you are being pulled in different directions learn to say no. Focus on what really matters.

Reward yourself: It takes effort and commitment to achieve your goal. Reward yourself each day for completing your tasks. It may be something small like meeting a friend for 15 minutes or a massage. These little rewards will pave the way for your continued success.

Magical 3: List 3 specific things you must do today to move you towards your goal. Every great journey is nothing more than a series of small steps taken in the right direction. Eventually you will arrive at your chosen destination. List these activities in order of importance and the challenge they present.

Secret 3: Feel Good Factors

The benefits of exercise can never be overstated. Exercise is one of the most positive methods of dissipating stress both physical and psychologically. Exercise releases a body's own feel good chemical called endorphins. It also reduces the build up of cortisol. Resistance training is one of the most beneficial ways to turn back the clock in the aging war. If you are feeling down, your body responds by producing cortisol. It is vital to seek professional help if it persists as it can be detrimental to your physical and mental wellbeing. Professional help will restore balance to your overall wellbeing.

Sense of purpose:

Each one of us is born with a life purpose. Most of us just amble along through life never addressing life's true purpose. You have been given talents which are truly unique to you. Identifying and pursuing this purpose is possibly the single most important action you can take to find fulfilment in your life. Take time to unravel the layers of misunderstanding, confusion and wrong decisions to discover what ignites your true passion! Find out what really motivates you. Without a sense of purpose in life, you can easily become distracted on your journey.

With a purpose, everything becomes clear. It simply means doing what you love. Once this is infused with clarity and enthusiasm, it is only a matter of time before you become an expert at it. By understanding your purpose, you are aligning yourself with your higher purpose which means others benefit also.

Social stimulation:

When you are confronted with negative energy, it can have a debilitating effect on you. Moods can alter. Choose individuals who will support and stimulate you. Volunteer for charity work; use your talents for others to benefit from.

The power of No:

The current demands that you are subjected to daily can leave you overwhelmed. As you struggle to meet the demands of your children, your partner and career it all take its toll. By prioritising your responsibilities you can manage your time more effectively and see what is really important. Learning how to say NO can be one of the most rewarding lessons you will ever learn. When you become exhausted the world takes on a different colour. The lines between personal and professional responsibilities become blurred as you struggle with so many demands in a desperate effort to please everyone. It is just as acceptable to say "no" as it is to say "yes" and you don't have to feel guilty!! You do not have to justify your actions.

Here are some examples of how you can reduce stress in you daily life:
1. Non-essential journeys - arrange for a pick up to take children to and from events, arrange with parents to do it in turns.
2. Non-essential e-mails such as jokes and spam. Write a polite email asking "to take you off the mailing list"
3. Prioritise your work load - don't become embroiled in other people's responsibilities. Insist that workers locate the relevant information required. If you permit yourself to become a shoulder to lean on, don't be surprised if it is abused.
4. Deadlines - ask to be notified in advance of deadlines as this will alleviate pressure. Politely advise co-workers what their responsibilities are and that last minute alterations are at their discretion.

Once you have identified how to prioritise your time and the art of delegation, look at other possibilities you can say "no" to.

Natural alternatives:

Switching from a toxic (manmade) to a more natural eating plan will have immediate positive results on your wellbeing. Eliminate all junk and fast food and notice significant improvements in your moods.

Limit alcohol consumption:

Your body metabolisms alcohol like fat, alcohol is essentially sugar in another form. Calories are extracted and stored around the mid section waiting to be used. Research has found that excess alcohol supports an increase of cortisol in your body making a flat, toned stomach virtually impossible to achieve. Have you ever wondered why men who guzzle beer have enormous paunches? The same rule applies to women who overindulge! It will leave an unsightly profile.

Alcohol has a negative effect not only on your fat burning abilities; it also hinders the use of vital minerals and vitamins in their unique roles. Vitamin B6 and calcium are particularly compromised. Excess alcohol also has a detrimental effect on your liver, heart and kidneys. It may lead to a number of serious ailments including cancer, pancreas disorders, mood swings and it can seriously affect your central nervous system. It can also be your ticket to depression. There is no question that it alters your physical and mental wellbeing. After a night of excess alcohol, you will crave junk food to replenish your energy levels and you will feel rotten, bloated and exhausted. If you wish to drink alcohol, organic wine is your safest bet with moderation as your key.

Lift weights:

The best possible prevention for osteoporosis is resistance training. Osteoporosis is the thinning of the bones which is more prevalent in women; vital vitamins like calcium diminish the density of the bone as you age, leaving it weaker and brittle with the passing of time. This condition may become chronic as it spreads throughout your body. Resistance training acts as a powerful anti-aging remedy.

Tips to prevent osteoporosis

- Do a resistance training workout three times per week.
- Also include a rich supply of calcium in your daily eating plan while ensuring you take vitamin C (1000 IU) and vitamin D (400 IU) daily.
- Try to maximise your sun exposure to a minimum of 15 to 30 minutes per day. Avoid the sun when it is at its strongest between 12 and 3 pm and always use sun protection.

14

The Most Commonly Asked Questions

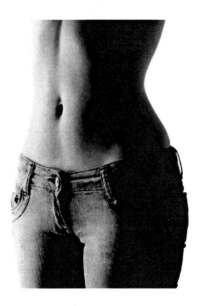

The "How to Get a Flat Stomach in 30 Days" eating plan and exercise routine are easy to follow but you may have questions about specific recommendations. This section will provide additional information in a question and answer format.

Can I eat rice and potatoes?

Rice and potatoes are excellent forms of carbohydrates which are packed with essential vitamins and minerals. Potatoes and rice are a high GI food which means they are absorbed quickly and released immediately into your blood stream. They elevate your blood sugars creating a spike which is quickly followed by a dip in your energy levels. These types of foods create an environment for highs and lows of your blood sugars. When you blood sugar hits a low patch you must refuel in an attempt to stabilise your blood sugar. This constant snacking on carbohydrates will manifest in weight gain. Try to eat them only at lunchtime.

Why is water so important?

Water has many health benefits and it acts as a detoxifying agent by flushing out the toxins out of your system. Water also acts as a cooling regulator carefully controlling your body's temperature. Taking 1 to 2 litres of water per day will keep your body hydrated while improving your concentration. Water also acts as a transporter of vital minerals and vitamins carrying them to their final destination.

What is a sensible weight loss target?

It is generally accepted that 2 pounds (0.9 Kg) of body fat per week is recommended. There are various factors which will influence the weight loss amount. Individual factors like your metabolic rate (the rate at which you burn calories), how active you are and how much weight you have to lose. The heavier you are - the faster you will respond to a balanced eating plan. On the flat stomach eating plan you will be eating 1200 calories and combined with your exercise routine this will give you a calorie deficit of 1000 per day. This will equate to 7000 calories per week which in turn means losing approx 1.5 to 2 pounds of body fat per week. Losing more weight than 2 pounds per week can usually be attributed to fluid loss. The first weeks are usually the most productive, as your body switches from a toxic eating plan to more natural eating plan. The results are immediate.

What about cheat meals?

The human body has been designed to desire sugar and salt. There is a rule which is absolutely written in stone: "What you eat you crave". Think for a moment about what you eat. Do you enjoy it? Reflect on this rule and identify what foods you crave. The artificial enhancing chemicals which make up a huge percentage of processed foods are there for a reason: so your taste buds will become addicted to these chemical agents.

Is it an accident that so many within our society have become addicted to this type of food? The fast food industry has made a fortune out of this type of addiction. Sugar and foods which contain it cause an overload of insulin and glucose in your system. If insulin is used immediately, it will cause the removal of fat from the blood stream and deposit it in fat cell storage. This has a cumulative effect of storing up unwanted glucose (sugar) around your mid section while waiting for it to be used as an energy source. Have the least amount of what you desire!

Is fast food and convenience food really that bad?

Yes, it is laden with artificial preservatives, synthetic fertilizers, pesticides and artificial flavouring to camouflage its lack of nutritional value. This type of food has one purpose: to make you gain weight and keep you coming back for more. The key question is how you feel after you have eaten a meal like this? If you feel bloated, uncomfortable and lethargic then you must resist this type of indulgence. The key is to return to food in its most natural state. This is how is how your body has been designed to function.

Almost all restaurant food comes pre-made, pre-mixed, frozen and in cans or containers. Most restaurants do not cook from scratch. The foods sold in fast food chains are laden with artificial flavouring to satisfy your taste buds and camouflage their lack of nutritional content. They often contain hydrogenated or partially hydrogenated oils and sweeteners such as aspartame. Meat and dairy products are loaded with growth hormones; antibiotics and other chemically enhancing agents which remove most of the nutritional value. The fast food outlets are quickly spreading their tentacles into every culture around the world. Always question where your food source originates from: Is it man made or natural?

Can I have fruit juices or diet drinks?

In your search for a solution to removing excess weight, processed fruit juices and diet drinks are problematic. Fruit juice is in many cases nothing more than sweetened water! Its nutritional goodness has been removed during the processing and sugar is substituted in an effort to satisfy your taste buds. This simple sugar is known as fructose, which after it has been absorbed into the bloodstream, goes directly to the liver where it metabolizes into fats called Triglycerides.

Diet drinks should be also avoided as they contain no nutritional benefits. Whatever traces of vitamins and minerals there might once have been in these drinks have been replaced with chemical agents to enhance flavouring. The best recommendation is to take natural fruit juice made of low glycaemic fruits which are less likely to promote weight gain.

I enjoy an alcoholic drink - what is the best choice?

Alcohol in moderation is acceptable; the best choice is organic wine. Alcohol is loaded with fructose. Once this is released into your blood stream it easily converts to sugar and if taken in excess will lead to weight gain. Alcohol will require the liver to work hard to process it, which diminishes your body's fat burning potential. If alcohol is off limits, it can have a negative physiological effect while struggling to adhere to the ban, you may find your will power challenged. In a nutshell, you must a solution that works for you. If that means having a limited amount of what you enjoy do it. Avoid beer as it is loaded with simple carbohydrates and is too easily converted into sugar by your body. Excess alcohol will increase your cortisol levels, the hormone which promotes fat accumulation around the mid section and butt. Allow 2 to 3 units of alcohol weekly.

Is organic always best?

The term organic is used to describe foods which have in grown in their natural habitat. It means foods which have been produced without the interference of chemically enhancing agents which unnaturally speed up the process of getting the product to your table. Organic produce remove the risk of consuming pesticides, fertilizers and growth hormones. Organic food is more expensive but it is worth it. You are investing in your most prized asset - yourself!

Can I substitute farmed fish, smoked meats or deli foods?

Nothing smoked, dried or chemically enhanced will replace organic food. The foods you choose must be of the leanest variety, remove all visible fats. All meat and fish should be organic otherwise it will contain growth hormones, antibiotics and other chemically enhancing agents which impair the fat burning process. Farmed fish are full of man-made chemicals with flavour enhancing chemicals which reduce the efficiency at which you remove fat.

Be very careful about using only grass fed beef and veal, otherwise you are likely to consume meat and poultry which have been fed on genetically modified grain and produce which result in a very high fat content.

Is Monosodium Glutamate (MSG) really that bad?

Yes. It should be avoided at all costs. It is packed with extremely dangerous toxins. It may increase depression and unnaturally increase your appetite. It has been shown to cause headaches and migraines and it also packs on the pounds!!

What if I miss meals?

Latest research has found that one of the main contributing factors linked to obesity is infrequent eating patterns. The human body has been designed to eat small meals regularly. The best type of food which can be digested easily is raw or unrefined food. Our bodies have adapted to our changing environment but they operate best by grazing. The human body is not well equipped to gorge followed by a fast of hours on end.

Are high-protein diets damaging?

There are many myths about protein. The truth is that like all foods, protein will generate metabolic waste which is released once it is dissolved with water. When consuming large amounts of protein it is crucial to drink plenty of water. This flushes the excess waste from your body. Remember protein is your building block for creating lean metabolically active muscle. When you cut calories, you body needs protein to prevent the metabolizing of muscle tissue to be used as an energy source. Protein will keep your energy levels high. An eating plan void of protein will produce a soft, shapeless appearance.

Can I skip breakfast?

One of the main causes for obesity has been found to be the eating of meals infrequently and consuming large amounts of foods at the wrong times. The human digestive system is designed to eat small meals every few hours and operates best by "grazing" on raw or unrefined foods. Thus, by skipping breakfast and eating a small lunch it is most likely you will consume a huge dinner at night. This places an unnatural burden on your digestive system allowing food which is consumed at night to be stored in fat deposit sites waiting to be used. In today's society, we often consume more food than is required - this food is easily digestible and often unrefined and floods the body with excess calories which are not required. The body must store these excess calories by creating fat deposit sites. This is why it has been medically proven that eating breakfast, lunch and a snack mid morning and mid afternoon followed by dinner no later than 6.30pm is the healthiest and best long term approaches for weight management and wellbeing.

What about fried, sauté and barbecue foods?

This type of food has been significantly altered from its original state by the cooking process. We are not biologically equipped to deal with type of altered food and the by-products of the cooking process remain undigested and assimilate a certain amount of residue in your body. This residue is toxic.

If this type of food dominates your eating plan, your digestive system will become overtaxed regularly. Your body is building up toxicity in two ways, through the normal process of the metabolising which takes place and by the residue left after certain foods which have not been effectively utilised. When toxic waste has not been removed, it will build up resulting in weight gain! Toxins are of acidic nature, when acid builds up in your body, your system retains water to neutralise it, resulting in bloating.

What about creams and pills which promise weight loss? Pills which reduce your appetite? Pills which increase your metabolic rate?

These products are mostly worthless! They do not work; they are a marketing tool to entice you to part with your hard earned cash. In some cases they may shift a few pounds temporarily due to some minor change in your eating plan but this is usually fluid or structural fat, and once you return to your original eating regime the pounds reappear. The only proven method for weight loss is a balanced eating plan combined with an exercise regime. If you want a flat stomach and to remove the excess fat from around your midsection you must follow the eating and exercising plan as outlined while customizing it to your life style. Don't waste your time searching for magic pills or potions – your wallet will thank you in the long term!

Are low fat foods ok?

Low fat foods are not necessarily low in calories. While manufactures may remove sugar from their products it is common practise to substitute the lack of sugar with artificial flavouring and other chemical additives to compensate. Some of these foods can disrupt your blood sugars and may promote fat being stored. It all comes down to calories in versus calories out. Foods with labels saying "low fat" or "Low carbohydrates" are usually marketing scams designed to deceive you. Always look for 100% organic.

What sauces can I use?

Use olive oil in moderation to enhance the flavour of your food. Sauces such as chilli and mustard sauces should be avoided where possible. Use spices or herbs to enhance the flavouring of foods, certain spices have been found to speed up the metabolism which in turn promotes weight loss.

How can I keep the weight off permanently?

If you go back to eating fast foods, processed foods, foods laden with Tran's fats, junk food and emotional eating with highly refined sugars and poor quality meats you will destroy your metabolism. If you follow the weight maintenance plan shown in this book then you will retain you desired results permanently.

Does my mental attitude play a role in weight loss?

You become what your dominate thoughts suggest. The pictures you hold of yourself in your mind have a powerful effect on your physiology and contribute to your overall success. One of the most effective techniques for achieving your goal of a flat stomach is to place a photo of exactly what you desire in your purse or wallet and visualize the desired outcome daily. This will help you programme your mind to create your desired outcome. Your dominating thoughts do become your reality.

My metabolism is slow, how can I speed it up?

Your "metabolism" is governed by your basal metabolic rate or (BMR). This is the rate at which energy is used to survive. It controls your internal functions such as your central nervous system, cardiac and respiratory systems. It also controls the activity of the secretion of hormones. Lean metabolically active muscle tissue is what sustains your metabolism functioning at a high level. Research has found that resistance training is the best way to increase your metabolism. The most metabolically active tissue is muscle. Research has found that you burn calories up to 48 hours after you finish a resistance programme.

I am hungry at night, how can I stop eating?

Eating at night is the most problematic habit which must be broken to ensure weight loss. Late eating promotes weight gain and obesity. Your metabolism shuts down at 6.30pm, food consumed after this goes into storage. Whatever calories consumed will be deposited around your midsection and butt!! By eating a large meal at 6.30 will ensure you do not get hungry. If you eat something light at 8pm (preferably protein based— nuts/yogurt) it

Does coffee have a negative effect on weight loss?

Coffee causes a "flight or fight" response. In this heightened sense, adrenaline is transported through your body sending a signal of panic; it raises your stress hormone levels and may inhibit nerve receptors sites. Your body responds by holding on to every calorie available. Avoid coffee if possible, if you really desire it, allow one cup daily.

Is fast food really that bad?

Yes, it is not food. It is combination of chemicals and sauces disguised with particles of poor quality meat designed to keep you coming back for more. It is highly addictive. This type of food is nutritionally barren. It is empty calories .It is usually prepared and precooked using the same formula. This type of food is usually loaded with salt and other flavouring which are of no benefit to you. Avoid fast food at all costs.

Is it vital to stick rigidly to the rules?

Yes, it is carefully structured and by eliminating one element of the eating plan may have disastrous consequences. If you are following the plan, but eat late at night you will gain weight. The core principles cannot be ignored. It takes 21 days for a new thought pattern to become established in your subconscious mind. Once a thought pattern is woven into your subconscious it adopts an automatic response. This is what is truly unique about this programme.

Do I have to do the exercise part?

Exercise plays a vital role in achieving our ideal weight and in retaining it, it also promotes wellness. Exercise releases endorphins which are your body's own feel good chemical. Exercise promotes anti-aging and decreases the risk of coronary or respiratory problems. If you are opposed to exercise, follow the food plan for 30 days. After include some form of exercise you enjoy for 30 to 40 minutes, four times per week.

What if I do only the eating plan?

The nutrition plan is the cornerstone of this programme. You will notice dramatic changes within days of embarking on the eating plan. Stick rigidly to the eating plan. You will notice the pounds disappear, no more bloating; your energy will improve as will your moods. One of the most interesting observations I have noticed is the increase in a person's self-confidence. The guiding principle is that you will gain weight by eating the wrong food, at the wrong time. By switching to fresh meat, fruit and vegetables and eating at the right time, you enable your body to function at its optimum level.

Organic food is expensive and I can't afford it. What should I do?

By choosing foods which are free of artificial flavouring and chemicals is the single most important thing you can do to lose weight and reach your target. Otherwise it will clog up your digestive leading you to a life of misery. You will never remove excess weight and keep it off permanently if you do not break the cycle now and choose sensibly. You are making the greatest investment with your hard earned cash!! You are investing in your greatest asset---- Yourself. Choose organic where possible.

I am going out for a meal, what should I do?

The most important principles when eating out are:
- Avoid the bread basket.
- Eat something light 30 minutes before you go out.
- Choose a fruit or soup starter.
- Fish or meat with steamed or raw vegetables for main course is preferable.
- Avoid desserts.
- One glass of wine is fine.
- Avoid white flour, potatoes, pasta and rice.
- Avoid fried foods.
- Stick to the low carbohydrate dishes & have water with lime which helps alkalinity in the blood stream and reduces the stress hormone cortisol.

I would love to exercise but I don't have the time?

You must prioritise and find the time. None of us have the time, but once you make it a top priority you will find a window which allows you to train 3 to 4 times per week. This excuse is usually a cop out. In over two decades of training people I never had one person say to me that they have too much time on their hands. We live in a hectic, fast paced world trying to juggle careers with family and it may leave you overwhelmed at times. I sympathize but do not condone. Find that window of opportunity that will allow you a little freedom, you will not regret it. Plan your day in advance so you can incorporate your training. If you feel you cannot do the full work out do half of it.

I have a layer of fat around my mid section that I cannot lose?

This is due to your carbohydrate intake. Eliminate heavy carbohydrates from your diet, increase your cardiovascular activity to 5 times per week working at a (If you are at the intermediate or advanced Level) 70%--80% of your maximum heart rate or 7—8 (R.P.E.) and remove any junk food from your diet. Try not to eat after 6.30 pm.

If I lift weights will I develop big muscles?

This question usually comes from women as they embark on a resistance programmed for the first time. Achieving large muscle mass is incredibly difficult, particularly for women as oestrogen will not permit it. You would have to train for years, consuming huge quantities of food combining a specific body building programme to get close to this. Resistance training is possibly the single most effective method of developing a lean, toned body.

I get bored with doing the same workout all the time?

I have a simple rule that I apply to my own workouts and those of my clients. I never repeat the same workout twice. Keep changing the format and exercises. Sometimes I will work very fast doing resistance training, sometimes very slow. Anything that will enhance your continuity and keeps up your enthusiasm works!

What If I miss a workout or if I break out on junk food?

Answer: The temptation is there for all of us. If you do break out or miss a workout the secret is to get back on track as quickly as possible. The most frustrating thing that can happen is if a client throws in the towel and reverts back to his old ways. One minor blip is not disastrous but to undo all of the work that has been achieved is disastrous. Do not go down the guilt road of self flagellation!! Get back on track immediately.

What if I give the programme a go and see what happens?

Answer: True change only comes from deep within, you must genuinely believe that you can and will change. If so follow the progression suggested above. You are challenging old belief patterns and infusing new beliefs which reflect your new self image. It is mandatory to truly believe you can and will achieve your desired weight and shape. This is what will motivate you in moments of despair should they arise. You must get the mental attitude correct, one of optimism replacing any old lingering self doubts. Be honest, if you wish to lose 60 pounds you will not achieve in 21 days! But you could in 6 or 7 months.

What is the best time to train?

Answer: Resent research suggests that training early in the day enhances continuity. You have your workout over and can face the day. If you leave your workout until night, there are a number of factors which may inhibit your session; meetings, an unexpected phone call, traffic or just worn out after a day's work may force you to miss your session.

Now that I am training can I eat junk because I will burn it off?

Answer: This is the rock you will perish on! Don't under any circumstances fall into this trap. At times with a new client when they are not progressing as quickly as I feel they should, I will sit down and ask them to come clean (knowing in advance what has happened) and invariably this is the answer. You may put weight on in this manner. NO JUNK! Apply the 90%--10% rule.

What is the most important meal of the day?

Answer: Research has found that breakfast is the most important meal of the day. It will allow your blood sugars to stabilise. After you have rested, you need an instant energy source. Fruit or oatmeal is the best choice. Recent studies have found that a common culprit for weight gain is eating irregularly and consuming massive meals late in the evening. The human body has been designed to graze throughout the day, eating every two and a half hours. The key is to consume the right type of food.

Why is sleep so important to weight loss?

Answer: During sleep, your body extracts the vitamins and minerals that it requires, when you wake up, usually you must visit the bathroom removing waste. Proper sleep will allow you to function efficiently, when sleep has been disturbed, it can leave you feeling drained.

Recent studies have found that people who have broken sleep or are tired need 30% more carbohydrate to sustain their energy levels than individuals who are not. Sleep naturally repairs the body's immune system or any ailment that can be restored without resorting to antibiotics. Sleep disorders may be caused by poor nutrition or eating late at night. Toxins or Trans fats may overload the digestive system, resulting in sleep deprivation. Exercise and three cups of camomile tea will assist in establishing proper sleeping patterns. Non prescription drugs should be avoided as they interfere with the natural sleeping cycle resulting in a dependency being formed.

What can I do to improve my mental and emotional wellbeing?

Answer: Physical exercise is the most important contribution you can make to improve your mental and emotional wellbeing. You will feel energised, positive and focused. Physical exercise is the single greatest investment of your time.

How can I prevent back pain?

Answer: Every year, the number of people who experience lower back pain increases. Surprisingly most people do not know what causes it. Back pain is often preventable, common examples include: being overweight may cause the lumbar spine to move out of its natural alignment or leaning forward to pick something up without bending your knees. Holding a heavy object away from your body will put a huge strain on your lumbar spine. If you experience a sharp pain in your lower back, immediately stop what you are doing. The sacro–iliac joint is easily thrown out of its natural position by sudden movements. Most experts agree that if back pain strikes, the worst thing you can do is to do nothing. Research has shown that people get better faster if they take gentle exercise.

The best methods of preventing back pain are:
- Swimming: but leave out the Brest stroke.
- Strengthen up the lower back.
- Losing weight.

It goes without saying that, when it comes to your back, all exercises must be done under the guidance of a trained professional.

Exercises for Strengthening the Back

1. Lie on the floor facing the ground. Allow your arms to lie by your side. Gently pull your upper body towards the ceiling. Hold at the top of the contraction for 10 seconds and return to your starting position. Repeat 5 times.
2. Once you are comfortable with this, the next stage is to put your hands on your temples and lift your upper body for a count of ten seconds. Repeat 5 times.
3. The last variation is to place your hands in the super man position (in front of you) and lifting yourself off the floor and holding for 10 seconds. Repeat 5 times.
4. Do a cat stretch and hold for 10 seconds at the end of your strengthening routine.

Is it ok to watch T.V. while eating?

No, if you are distracted while eating, you may over indulge.

Why do I not lose weight permanently on a diet?

Here is a list of 10 reasons why you will not lose weight on a diet permanently.

1. Shock to the system

When you body is deprived of food, it goes into a state of shock. In this state, your body holds onto every calorie possible. With the looming prospect of a famine, it refuses to burn calories.

2. No exercise

Most diets do not highlight the importance of exercise. Cardiovascular exercise will speed up your metabolism, and help in burning calories. Resistance exercises will also speed up your metabolism while toning the desired areas.

3.   Processed foods

While you attempt to wean yourself off processed foods, the chemical components of this type of food may lead to withdrawal symptoms, instead of going cold turkey, a gradual removal of this type of food is more desirable. If it is too drastic, it may leave you feeling miserable and despondent.

4.   Boredom

Consuming the same type of bland food will soon become irritating. In order to be successful you must establish an eating plan which is realistic and enjoyable or failure is just around the corner.

5.   Expense

Some diets can insist on a variety of supplements and expensive foods. This is short circuiting the natural process. It is unnecessary.

6.   Severe

Many diets can be so severe that they are unrealistic. Like not eating for hours on end, taking only shakes etc. This will lose fluid, but it is unrealistic. How long can you survive like this?

When you have an addiction for certain types of chemical foods, you have an addiction to the chemicals in this food, when you go cold turkey and completely remove this type of food from your eating plan, you go through withdrawals!! A gradual removal of this type of food is more sustainable.

7.   Banishing the foods you love

You have your vices, things you love. If you remove them altogether from your life, what will be the likely outcome? By applying the 90/10 rule you can still enjoy what you love but in moderation. This in turn will enhance your continuity and your chances of developing an eating plan that you can successfully incorporate into the rest of your life. It physiologically improves your mental wellbeing.

8. Holidays

After your hard work, you finally go on that much deserved holiday. The moment you come off a diet and indulgence, the weight comes back faster than ever. This can have a detrimental effect. You feel bloated and disillusioned. You need to have a measured and realistic approach to your eating habits. The weight maintenance programme allows you to eat sensibly and enjoy yourself.

9. Incorrect food combining

By applying the simple techniques of proper food combining, you will feel energised and not bloated. Remember the last time you felt bloated? It is terrible.

10. Empty calories

Diets which allow you to consume empty calories will leave you malnourished and hungry. It is not a sensible approach.

What is the most effective anti aging and overall wellness programme?

These are the most important factors.
*   4 to 6 carrots and 2 apples per daily (in smoothies if you prefer)
*   Avoid coffee and processed foods, junk and take away foods
*   9 hours sleep each night
*   2 litres of water every day
*   Herbal teas taken every day
*   Eat plenty of salmon, melon and fruit
*   Vitamin C - 1000.iu per day
*   Vitamin E - 400iu per day
*   Use the eating plan shown in chapter 8
*   Adhere to the above and exercise 3 to 4 times per week, incorporating both resistance and cardiovascular exercises.

Is it possible to prevent cancer by eating certain foods?

You can reduce the chances of getting cancer by making certain changes to your eating plan. Latest research indicates that consuming a wide variety of different coloured fruits and vegetables daily can help in preventing cancer. Smoothies are a convenient way to do this. Also follow the advice in this list:

Do's
- Consume 3 cups of green tea daily.
- Plenty of fresh fruit and vegetables daily.
- Soya products daily are desired.
- Linseed is highly recommended by the National Cancer Institute.
- Green vegetables are excellent antioxidant.
- White meat is desirable.
- Stay as close to natural foods as possible.
- Wild fish daily.
- Berries are an excellent source of Antioxidants.
- 2 litres of water per day helps to keep you hydrated, while flushing out toxins.

Do Not's
- Don't eat red meat more than twice a week.
- Don't eat processed foods.
- Don't consume foods cooked in vegetable oil.
- Don't smoke.
- Don't consume take away foods.
- Don't consume precooked foods.
- Don't consume foods laden with artificial sauces.
- Don't eat junk.
- Don't consume more than 2-3 units of alcohol per week.

An eating plan which follows the above advice can reduce the chances of contracting cancer as it is loaded with antioxidants. Proper nutrition is emerging key for cancer prevention. The real secret is to stay as close to nature as possible.

What is the best way to beat that afternoon slump?

Recent findings show that the most common time for your energy levels to slump is between 2.30 and 4.00 pm. It may leave you feeling drained and difficult to concentrate. If you suffer a dip in your energy mid afternoon, try a few of these tips to restore it.

Do's
- Have a piece of fruit.
- Have a handful of non salted nuts.
- Have a cup of herbal tea.
- Have a short break in the fresh air.
- Have a glass of water every hour.
- Have a light lunch & food combine correctly.

Do Not's
- Don't have a heavy meal at lunch.
- Don't eat chocolate or pastries.
- Don't drink coffee.
- Don't drink alcohol at lunch.
- Don't overstress yourself, prioritise your work.
  Don't eat salted foods.
  Don't eat fried foods at lunch.

What is the best training programme for building muscle?

A programme I discovered is the 6x6 programme. You choose a weight that you can just about do 6 reps with, allow yourself 30 seconds rest and then repeat 6 times. Choose 3 different exercises for one body part. Take the chest, do 6 sets of 6 reps on the bench press followed by 6 sets of 6 reps on the incline press and lastly do 6 sets of 6 reps on the dips. You may use 30 seconds rest between each set. Do one body part per day. After 3 to 4 weeks you can superset the exercises like chest and back, biceps and triceps where you do 6 sets of 6 exercises for chest and back. So it would be a set of bench press immediately followed by a set of pull ups, then rest for 30 seconds. Take 3 exercises and super 6x6 using the above formula. You must have being training for at least 6 months before you do this programme.

Is it possible to eat yourself happy?

Serotonin is the happy hormone which is stored in your brain. It enables you to feel good about yourself, happy and relaxed. When you remove certain foods from your daily eating plan, it may result in you feeling miserable and may be a factor in headaches and irritable bowel syndrome. If this is not corrected over a period of time it can result in depression.

It is now known that reducing a variety of carbohydrates foods will affect you negatively. The key is to know which carbohydrates will create that feel good factor and which will not. A common mistake is to try to remove all carbohydrates form your eating plan in the attempt to lose weight quickly. This may leave you miserable, tired and irritable. The secret is that eating a wide range of natural foods will increase your serotonin levels and improve your overall wellness.

Which foods offer such benefits? Avoid white flour, processed foods and chemically made food. This type of food will give you a sudden burst of energy followed by a sudden drop in energy. Wise choices are natural carbohydrates and proteins. They will fill you up and also supply you with the necessary vitamins and minerals needed. Whole grain brown bread, non salted nuts, brown pasta, and organic dairy products are ideal. They will also minimise the effects of stress and enable you to sleep better. Eating high protein natural foods will also boost your serotonin levels, cheese, white meat and eggs are ideal. Other foods which will increase your serotonin levels are bananas and avocado pears. Eat plenty of raw fresh fruit and vegetables.

If you feel persistently tired, your iron levels may be low, so readjust your eating plan to include red meat twice a week, eggs, nuts, leafy green vegetables such as spinach and liver are all excellent ways to boost your iron levels. Calcium is one of the most effective mood enhancers which are found in dairy products, choose natural dairy produce. Magnesium will repair the muscle tissue with speedy results; also it helps you to remain relaxed. Green leafy vegetables, wild fish, seeds and almonds nuts are excellent sources of magnesium.

The message is that with all of the bad press that carbohydrates have received, you need the right type of carbohydrates and protein to lose weight effectively and support your overall happiness.

Before you eat anything, ask yourself how is this food made? Is it natural or has it been made by man with a combination of chemicals and flavouring? Once you choose natural products you are on the right path. Another common mistake to losing weight is to starve yourself in the belief that the pounds will disappear. This will only lead you to becoming sick and drained of energy.

Serotonin boosters:

- Fruit and vegetables
- Brown wholemeal bread, brown pasta and wild rice
- Garlic
- Bananas

What is the Rainbow Eating Plan?

For a more radiant-looking you, take a look at what you can achieve by following the rainbow eating plan. It may be taken in smoothies if you prefer.

Red = Smooth skin
An eating plan rich in the powerful antioxidant Lycopene will help you to look fabulous. Lycopene can be found in tomatoes, watermelon, papaya and red grapefruit. It also is a powerful anti-cancer agent that helps to prevent cell anti-aging.

Purple = Wrinkle free
One of the most powerful skin boosting antioxidants identified by resent research is anthocyanin, which keeps skin firm and young looking. It may be found in blueberries, beetroot and red grapes.

Green = Banish Cellulite
Asparagus, broccoli, spinach are great sources of folic acid, the B vitamin which supports your overall health and wellbeing. It helps to encourage the body's cells to release toxins.

Orange = Clear eyes
If you wish to enhance the brightness of your eyes, beta-carotene is a wonderful natural remedy. Carrots, apricots and mangoes contain high levels of beta-carotene. Another tip is to never work in a darkened room at the computer.

151

White = Weight loss
A proper digestive system will enhance your energy. Leeks, onions and shallots will support good bacteria in your stomach. Organic yogurt or a live probiotic drink will stimulate healthy bacteria, preventing illness.

Brown = Healthy heart
Wholemeal bread, brown rice and seeds are an excellent source of fibre and energy. They provide both vitamin B and minerals.

Yellow = Great hair
As you grow older, your hormone levels drop which may result in thinning or dry hair. Yellow foods are a wonderful source of antioxidants and also have regenerating benefits and overall health wellbeing properties. Bananas, yogurts, pumpkin seeds are ideal.

The Three Day Anti Aging Formula

Breakfast
Glass of warm water with fresh lemon
Chose one of the following
- Bowl of fresh fruit(melon/berries/apple/pineapple)
- Oatmeal with selection of fresh berries
- Fruit smoothies (three oranges and one lemon)

11 am
A cupful of non salted nuts

Lunch
Two glasses of water
Choose from one of the following
- White organic meat salad/olive oil/tomatoes/olives
- Grilled wild fish/brown rice/olive oil/basil dressing/green beans
- Cottage cheese salad
- Bowl of homemade soup and a slice of wholemeal brown bread

4 pm
Banana

Dinner
Eat a large meal
Chose one of the following
- Grilled meat/spinach/olive oil/vegetables of your choosing
- Wild salmon with a selection of green vegetables
- Roasted vegetables with pine nuts mixed through

Supper
Chose one of the following
- Glass of apple and carrot juice freshly squeezed (6 carrots and 2 apples)
- Slice of melon and a cupful of berries mixed in organic yogurt
- Non salted nuts mixed in with organic yogurt
- Cup of green tea and a slice of melon

Things you should do
- Get 9 to 10 hours rest per night
- Drink 2 glasses of water with each meal
- Do not eat a heavy meal after 6.30 pm
- Take in plenty of fresh berries and melon daily
- Allow one cup of coffee per day if you really require it
- Choose fresh fruit and vegetables where possible
- Choose organic food
- Take in 2 to 3 units of dairy products per day (unit is the size of a cup)
- Take vitamin C 1000 iu and vitamin E 400 iu daily
- Take protein at night, yogurt with non salted nuts mixed in

Things you should not do
- Eat foods which contain white flour
- Eat foods which contain trans fats
- Eat take away foods
- Eat fast foods
- Eat processed foods

15

The Flat Stomach Guide to Staying Slim

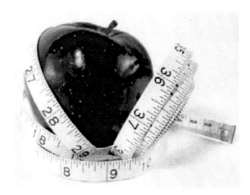

The 90/10 Rule

We can learn a lot about nutrition from books, some suggest taking a vow of junk food abstinence. Is this realistic? If you have a ban on your favourite treat, this may result in craving it even more. This is often followed by a binge resulting in overeating and then feeling rotten and demoralised that you have failed. The solution is to engage in an eating plan that you can stick with for the rest of your life. Consistency is the hall mark of a successful eating and exercise routine. Physiologically clients are much stronger when you factor in a reward system. It takes hard work and dedication to lose weight and maintain your ideal weight, allowing for a reward comes with guidelines. The basic rule" Eat the least amount you will get away with". Do not eat late at night and you must eat some form of protein 30 minutes before you indulge.

The way this rule works is, you should aim to eat healthy and exercise 90% of the time. Allow yourself to indulge 10% of the time. This allows you to enjoy yourself making everything worthwhile, incorporating new rules into your lifestyle. Do not allow yourself to slip back into old eating habits. Apathy will cause weight gain. If you crave something, have just enough to satisfy your craving. Otherwise you will make yourself miserable.

Guidelines for Proper Eating

1. Use fresh fruit and vegetables whenever available
2. Eat fruit when hungry - 30 min before or after a meal
3. Use olive oil as dressing
4. Avoid vinegar in dressing
5. Use only whole-grain breads
6. Drink juice on empty stomach not immediately following any other food.
7. Use proper food combining
8. Do not overeat, use proper portion sizes

The Energy Ladder

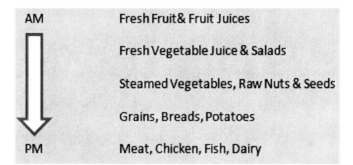

AM	Fresh Fruit & Fruit Juices
	Fresh Vegetable Juice & Salads
	Steamed Vegetables, Raw Nuts & Seeds
	Grains, Breads, Potatoes
PM	Meat, Chicken, Fish, Dairy

The energy ladder is shown in the box above and shows the time of day when certain foods should be eaten. Foods high in natural sugars and carbohydrates should be eaten early in the day (such as fruit juices) while protein rich foods (such as meats and dairy) should be eaten towards the end of the day.

Breakfast Guidelines

- Start the day with fresh fruit or oatmeal with berries mixed through it.
- Eat fruit throughout the morning.
- Fruit must be fresh no concentrated juices or juices "made from concentrate".
- The correct time to consume fruit is 30 min before or after a meal

Weight Maintenance Plan

Once you have achieved your desired weight or body shape you should start to increase carbohydrate intake to 3 to 4 units per day.

Breakfast
Chose from one of the following
- Poached eggs with mushrooms and tomatoes
- Oatmeal
- Scrambled eggs with one slice of whole meal brown bread
- Fruit with nuts mixed through

11 am
A piece of fruit of your choosing

Lunch
Chose from one of the following
- Whole meal brown bread salad sandwich
- Bowl of minestrone soup with one slice of wholemeal bread
- Cottage cheese salad

4 pm
A cupful of non salted nuts

Dinner
Choose from one of the following
- Baked sea bass on a bed of lentils and green beans
- Stir fried vegetables (olive oil) with goats cheese mixed through
- Avocado prawn salad using olive oil if necessary
- Monk fish with green beans

Supper
Choose from one of the following
- Allow 2 oat meal biscuits with a cup of green tea
- Organic yogurt with non salted nuts mixed through
- Carrot and apple juice (freshly squeezed)

Things you should do
- Never allow yourself to get hungry

- Eat every two hours
- Keep food as close to its natural state as possible
- Avoid foods laden with salt
- Never eat large meals after 6.30 pm
- Keep yourself hydrated (2 litres of water daily)
- Avoid junk and fried foods
- Limit caffeine to one cup per day
- Avoid take away food
- Take in 2 to 3 units (cup full) of dairy products daily

The Flat Stomach 5 Rules for Success

Rule one: Allow two units of carbohydrate per day along with your eating plan.

Rule two: No junk.

Rule three: No eating after 6.30 with the exception of something light.

Rule four: Two litres of water per day.

Rule five: You crave what you eat. Choose foods which are as close to their natural state as possible.

16

100 Flat Stomach Boosters

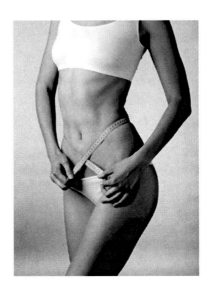

Things you must do.

1. Choose organic food.
2. No eating after 6.30 pm, except something light.
3. Less calories going in with more calories going out equals a calorie deficit.
4. No junk & two litres of water per day.
5. Eat 3 to 5 pieces of fruit per day.
6. Eat fresh vegetables every day.
7. Use proper food combining.
8. Avoid processed foods.
9. Exercise 4 times per week for approx 40 minutes.
10. Eat foods as close to their natural state as possible.
11. No microwaving.
12. Take one or two smoothies per day.
13. Choose an exercise program you enjoy.
14. Set weekly targets and reward yourself.
15. Change your exercise regime daily.

16. Rest, get 8 to 9 hours sleep per night
17. No fast food.
18. Get fresh air daily.
19. Take 30 minute power naps three times per week.
20. Eat pumpkin seeds daily.
21. Sleep well.
22. Take Vitamin D daily.
23. Don't use computers in a dark room, switch on the lights.
24. Stretch out daily.
25. Take non salted nuts daily.
26. Eat one banana a day.
27. Be positive and focus on your goals
28. Find a exercise you enjoy and apply the structure to it
29. Educate yourself about natural foods

Things you should do.

30. Eat some form of protein at night (non salted nuts).
31. Limit caffeine to one cup per day.
32. Choose herbal teas.
33. Have one cup of green tea per day.
34. Never skip breakfast.
35. Resistance training 3 times per week.
36. Cardiovascular training 3 times per week.
37. Use a steam room.
38. Wean yourself off sugar.
39. Take Vitamin C (1000 IU capsule per day)
40. Take fish oils supplements if you do not like fish.
41. Get 60 minutes of sunlight per day.
42. Consume carbohydrates at midday.
43. Snack on fresh fruit or non salted nuts.
44. Eat every two and half hours.
45. Avoid beer.
46. Choose wine if you wish to have a drink.
47. Drink only filtered water.
48. Have a Jacuzzi twice per week.
49. Take oatmeal daily.
50. Take flaxseed in the morning.
51. Take only whole meal brown bread (2 slices per day).
52. Pasta twice per week (Use a tomato base and have it at lunch time)
53. Choose brown wild rice, instead of white rice.
54. Reward yourself for reaching your short term goals.

Eight miracle foods which you should eat daily

55. Oatmeal
56. Organic fruit
57. Nuts
58. Organic Yogurt
59. Organic fish or meat
60. Green vegetables
61. Berries
62. Tomatoes

Things you should <u>not</u> do

63. Do not allow yourself to get run down
64. Do not consume preheated meals
65. Do not use artificial sweeteners
66. Do not use non prescription drugs
67. Do not consume refined sugar
68. Do not consume white flour
69. Do not eat cakes or scones
70. Do not eat Jam
71. Do not take any growth hormones
72. Do not use any powered substance which promote weight loss
73. Do not use any stimulus that artificially enhances your work outs

Things you must not do.

74. Do not eat fast food
75. Do not eat convenience food
76. Do not eat microwave food
77. Do not eat late at night
78. Do not snack on junk food
79. Do not eat take away oriental food
80. Do not eat monosodium glutamate (MSG)
81. Do not use sauces apart from olive oil
82. Do not eat anything that contains refined white flour
83. Do not eat anything that contains sugar
84. Do not eat any man made food
85. Do not eat anything that contains trans fat
86. Do not eat smoked or barbequed foods

87. Do not eat pickled foods
88. Do not eat anything that contains artificial sweeteners
89. Do not eat toxic food
90. Do not eat ice cream
91. Do not eat pizza
92. Do not eat gravy
93. Do not eat meat or fish which has been chemically modified
94. Do not eat farmed fish
95. Avoid foods which are "low fat" or "light"
96. Do not food combine incorrectly
97. Do not use salt
98. Do not drink tap water – buy bottled water
99. Do not drink fizzy drinks
100. Do not use sun beds.

Weight Gain – The Causes

As well as giving you the 100 tips above, I want to give you a simple list that gives you causes of gaining weight. If you need motivation, take a look at this list and see the reasons why you gained weight in the first place:

- Toxic food
- Junk food
- Snacking on junk
- Emotional eating
- Binge eating
- Late night eating
- Huge amounts of food being consumed at night
- Underactive thyroid gland
- Underactive metabolism
- Infrequent eating patterns
- Tiredness
- Stress
- Pressure
- Emotional upsets
- Low self esteem
- Poor self image
- Food addictions
- Blocked intestine
- Food which is nutritionally barren
- Consuming empty calories
- Low fat foods
- No exercise

17

Dying to be Golden

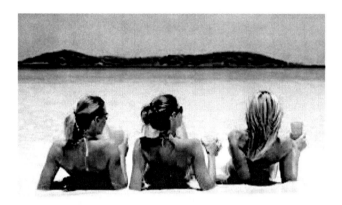

Follow a Few Simple Safety Rules to Protect You and Your Family from Skin Cancer

Once you have achieved your flat stomach, what better way to reward yourself than showing it off! A holiday lounging around in the summer sunshine will work wonders for recharging your batteries and improving your self-esteem. Feeling those rays on your tender skin is one of life's most cherished gifts. But reckless sunbathing can have serious consequences. It has been clearly proven that sunburn greatly increases the risk of developing skin cancer. Last year in Great Britain 100,000 cases of skin cancer were diagnosed.

What about indoor tanning? Steven Q. Wang, MD, is a member of the skin cancer foundation's independent photobiology committee and director of dermatologic surgery and dermatology at a large hospital in New Jersey. When examining recent research results Dr. Wang stated that "While the medical community has known anecdotally that indoor tanning is linked with melanoma (skin cancer), it has been difficult to provide the evidence. These new studies show conclusively that indoor tanning bed use can lead to melanoma". There is no little doubt in the scientific community that indoor tanning machines are a very bad idea!

Protect yourself.

The overwhelming advice is that skin cancer is avoidable; taking simple steps will ensure your safety and enjoyment of the sun. It is perfectly safe and natural for most people to enjoy the sun in moderation. Sunburn causes 85% of melanoma cases, so avoid sunburn at all costs. We are all at risk from skin cancer, but learn to be aware of the early warning signs.

It may obvious, but using sun screen is possibly the best protection if you want to tan safely. The stronger the factor the more protection it will offer. Application is the key: research has shown that correct application may reduce the chances of contacting skin cancer by 50%.

In a recent study carried out in Australia over 15 years, researchers divided their 1600 subjects into two groups, one applying sunscreen every day and the other only when they thought it was necessary. Both groups followed their patterns for five years and were monitored by researchers for a further ten years. The results, published in the Journal of Oncology, showed that 11 of participants in the first group developed malignant melanoma, compared to 22 cases in the second group who applied sunscreen only when necessary. Two of 11 melanomas diagnosed in the group who used daily sunscreen were severe, but in the second group 11 out of the 22 were severe. These finding came as no surprise to Dr. Nick Lowe, one of the UK's leading dermatologists. "I have always advocated daily sunscreen use" he says "both to reduce skin cancer and slow the visible signs of aging"

Nine Safe Sun Tanning Tips

Many women, and even some men, will do just about anything to get that perfect tan. But, with so much news about skin cancer and other problems associated with overexposure to the sun, many are wondering how to still get that great tan, while avoiding the potential side effects of sunbathing.

Safe Tanning Tip 1

Always wear sun block! With a sun block with a low SPF, your body can still catch some of the sun's rays, but you are less likely to get burned. A tan is basically your body's way of protecting itself from the harmful effects of the sun. The more you can slow down this process, the less your skin will receive long-term damage from sunbathing.

Safe Tanning Tip 2

You should gradually build up the time you spend in the sun. Many people are tempted to intentionally burn themselves right away, believing this provides a good "base" for the tan. Sunburns are a sign of skin damage and can lead to serious skin complications. Instead, the tan should be slowly built up to lessen the potential damage.

Safe Tanning Tip 3

You should apply your sun block to your body before you head out to the sun. Applying sun block first helps ensure that you get cover your entire body, guaranteeing that all of your skin is protected. And don't forget to apply sun block to your lips! Lips can become easily burned or dried out, which is both unhealthy for your skin and unattractive.

Safe Tanning Tip 4

The sun is at its hottest between noon and 3:00. Avoid sunbathing at this time. The added intensity of the sun does not improve the look of your tan. Instead, it increases you likelihood of becoming burned and, consequently, experiencing skin damage. During this time of the day, it is best to stay in a shaded area and to wear protective clothing.

Safe Tanning Tip 5

Spending time in the water increases your chances of getting sunburned. The sun's rays reflect from the water and are basically magnified onto your body. Getting sunburn while in the water can happen with little to know warning signs. Where a sun block, even if it is a low SPF, every time you are in water. Make sure the sun block is water resistant, as well, and reapply it as often as the product recommends. This is normally at least every 2-3 hours.

Safe Tanning Tip 6

Hats and shirts do provide an extra layer of protection to your skin. Be sure to wear these when not sunbathing in order to protect your skin from excessive amounts of sun. This is particularly important if you will be spending a great deal of time outdoors, such as playing sports or gardening.

Safe Tanning Tip 7

If you do play a lot of sports or if you work outdoors and sweat a great deal, be sure to wear a sun block that is specially formulated for such activities. Waterproof sun blocks are ideal for those who are active during the day outdoors.

Safe Tanning Tip 8

People with fair skin need to be especially cautious when exposing their skin to the sun for long periods of time. The same is true for people who burn easily or who have a history of tanning poorly. People with freckles or a great number of moles should also take extra precautions when spending time in the sun. People who fit under any of these categories are at a greater risk of developing skin cancer. Similarly, children under the age of 16 and individuals with a family history of skin cancer should avoid exposing their skin to excessive amounts of sun.

Safe Tanning Tip 9

If you have sensitive skin, make sure to purchase a sun block that will not irritate your skin. There are hypoallergenic sun block's available. If you are not sure where to look or what you need for your skin, ask the pharmacist and she will be glad to help.

18

Flat Stomach Forever – Rules to Live By

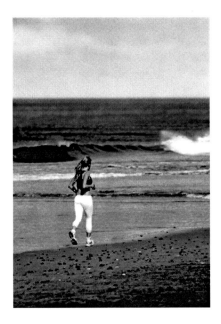

A Changed Lifestyle

Now that you have achieved your ideal weight and a flat stomach, you must make lifestyle choices to maintain your new shape. Unless you mentally adjust and put in place a maintenance plan you will join the long list of unsuccessful dieters who struggle with their weight all of their lives. By making small lifestyle changes you will maintain your ideal shape for the remainder of your life.

It is an unfortunate fact that 90% of dieters regain the weight they lost while following the diet. After finishing a weight loss regime, the weight which is regained is fatty tissue which is deposited at sites around your body (mostly the stomach & thighs). This new fatty tissue alters your body's composition making it even more difficult to lose this new weight. In order to avoid this happening, follow this step by step approach:

Step 1: Weight maintenance adaption

Readjust your eating plan to move into weight maintenance mode. This will allow you more variety to your eating plan while ensuring your weight stabilises at its correct level. Studies have shown that individuals who have successfully maintained their ideal weight have made lifestyle choices which have enabled them to retain their ideal shape. It all boils down to "calories in versus calories out". If the weight begins to creep back, go back to the original eating plan while increasing you physical activity.

Step 2: No eating after 6.30pm (except small amounts of protein)

This rule is written in stone. Food consumed after 6.30 pm will be deposited around your mid-section and thighs. If possible, consume the bulk of your food before 6.30pm; remember to eat a large meal at 6.30 as it will ensure you do not get hungry later. If you feel hungry, eat some form of protein (non salted nuts, cottage cheese or organic yogurt) before going to bed.

Step3: Remember that "what you eat you crave"

Your daily plan composition should be 40% carbohydrates, 30% fat and 30% protein. Whatever you eat, your taste buds will adjust and crave this particular type of food. We are prisoners of our taste bud. We will do anything to satisfy their needs. Many times you will eat foods which taste good, and then clog up your body, ensuring weight gain. It is important to eat foods that you enjoy but also meet the requirements of your body. The more healthy food that you eat – the more your taste buds and body will desire healthy food.

Step 4: Be active - be alive

Our bodies have evolved through millions of years of evolution to be efficient movers. We are basically designed to move around and to get exercise every day. We are not designed to laze about on a couch in front of a TV or sit in front of a computer all day! By adhering to an exercise regime, you are using the most effective weight maintenance tool at your disposal. Not only will exercise stabilise your weight but it will also improve your self-esteem and emotional wellbeing. The release of endorphins (the bodies own feel good chemical) will enhance your moods and physical changes to your appearance will increase your self confidence. Everything in your life revolves around your self esteem. This is the key to lasting change. As your self esteem becomes stronger you can channel this new found energy into any aspect of your life. Individuals who have relapsed and regained the weight they lost, tend to have a low self-image. They expect failure.

When you exercise you will:
- automatically will choose the right type of foods, as your body will crave them.
- feel and look better.
- improve your cardiovascular fitness.
- improve your muscle tone.

In order to maintain your ideal weight, you should aim to exercise 4 times per week for approximately 45 minutes. This should be a combination of resistance training and cardiovascular training. Research has found that a combination of resistance training and cardiovascular training is most effective for burning calories. Recommended choices: Power walking, Aerobic classes, Resistance training, swimming and jogging.

Step 5: Water, Water, Water!

As an absolute prerequisite to life, water is at the top of the list. From the moment you were born until the moment you leave this planet your body instinctively craves food, water, air and shelter for its survival. Your body is made up of 70% water. Water regulates your body's temperature while flushing harmful toxins out of your system.

Most people these days do not drink enough water and are effectively dehydrated all the time! If you feel tired, dizzy and grouchy a lot of the time then it is likely you are dehydrated. These are the early signs that you are not getting enough water. While the thing we most associate most with dehydration is feeling thirsty, in actual fact this doesn't happen until later. A recent study undertaken by Kings College London revealed that even mild thirst can decrease productivity at work by as much as 10%. Furthermore, hand to eye co-ordination can weaken at just one per cent dehydration. The good news is that dehydration can be rectified quickly. When scientists from the college of Institute of Psychiatry examined the effects of dehydration, they found that 90 minutes of sweating caused their subjects brains to shrink as much as a year of ageing, forcing them to work harder than brains not affected by dehydration. However, once the subjects were hydrated, their brains soon returned to normal.

As a general guideline you should drink 8 to 10 glasses of water daily:
- Switch from the caffeine-rich coffee to a glass of distilled water.
- If you find the flavour of water plain, add some lemon or blackcurrant.
- Place a large bottle of water at your desk or kitchen to remind you to consume 8-10 glasses of water daily.
- Consume water rich foods like melon or water melon daily.

One word of caution: do not drink a lot of water with a meal. If large quantities of water are taken with a meal, it impedes the efficiency of the digestive process. The digestive juices required to break down food become diluted resulting in the meal not being properly digested. Instead, spread your water consumption out throughout the day.

Step 6: Correct fruit consumption

Fruit has been found to be, without question, the most important food we can put into our bodies. It is imperative for your body to be cleansed of toxicity. The most effective cleansing agent is water rich foods. Fruit has been found to have the highest water content of any food. The body's requirements of protein, carbohydrates, fats, minerals and amino acids can all be found in fruit. Fruit has been hailed as the most perfect food source available with no other foods matching its benefits. When fruit is consumed correctly, eaten either before or after a meal, no other food source can replicate its cleansing or life giving benefits. As a tool for weight loss or weight management, the proper consumption of fruit remains unchallenged. You should aim to consume 3 to 5 pieces of fruit daily.

Final Word

There is an innate quality deeply embedded in the human psyche, we are always striving for what we cannot have, once we have what we dearly wanted, it loses its appeal. We are constantly looking for new challenge. The key is to know what you have and cherish it. There is an old Irish saying "The grass always seems greener on the other side of the hill, but it seldom ever is". Lasting change only comes from an eating and exercise plan that you enjoy. Once you have identified this, apply the structure that you have learnt and incorporate it into your daily life.

This book covers a huge amount of material about weight gain, weight loss, exercise and wellness. You have in your hand a book which will literally change your life in 30 days and you will never look back. The changes you will experience are profound, both physically and psychologically. The information in this book has taken years to research; it is backed up by leading experts. I personally guarantee that if you do the programme for 30 days, staying rigidly to the format, that you will be astonished by the results. As you change from a toxic eating plan to a natural eating regime, the results are miraculous. My sole motivation for writing this book is to share with you a winning formula for weight loss. It has dramatically improved my life as it will do for you.

Weight loss is a complex issue and it is important to understand what caused it to happen to you. It is about confronting your obstacles, whether they are: emotional eating or poor nutrition or an underperforming metabolism and finding the correct formula for you. Identify each step of the MERC strategy that works for you and customise it. Find your role model and identify exactly what you want. Change your self-image; until you sever the links with the old image you cannot embrace the new one. Your old self image will keep you imprisoned with how you saw yourself; it will keep producing the same results. I cannot stress the importance of developing the correct mental attitude, of having a deep down belief that you will achieve your heart's desire. This belief makes all the effort worthwhile. Knowing you are on the road to achieving your dream is an incredible feeling. I know because I achieved mine, now it is your turn. Always keep changing your eating plan and exercise regime, keep it interesting and enjoy the process. The single biggest threat to your success is that switch on your mind; always keep it in the on position. Enjoy what you are doing. Once the enjoyment goes out of it, is only a matter of time before you throw in the towel. Constantly reward yourself by setting daily goals and reward yourself for your accomplishment. You need hope and purpose in your life. Hope is like oxygen breathing life into your dreams, you cannot live without hope.

Learn to trust that inner voice which is guiding you, if you feel bad about something you are moving out of harmony with your life's mission. Trust your intuition and follow its path, if you feel good about something you are aligning yourself with your higher purpose. Inner peace is the result of trusting your inner judgment and acting on its guidance. Working on your mental and physical wellbeing is paramount for a happy life.

One final gem to leave you with: keep a written food diary. It will only take a moment to fill out but it is indispensible. It keeps you firmly focused on your goal.

You can break free from the shackles of excess weight once and for all. You will never have to go on a diet again. You have the power to shape your life and live it exactly how you want to. Do It!

Wishing you health, happiness and nothing but success.

Kevin Sheridan
August 2011

Appendix 1

Useful Recipes

French dressing:

Makes about 120ml/ 4fl oz/ 1/2cup

Ingredients:

90ml/ 6 tbsp extra virgin olive oil
15ml/ 1 tbsp white wine vinegar
5ml/ 1tsp French mustard
Pinch of caster sugar

Method

Measure the extra virgin olive oil and white wine vinegar into a small screw-jar-top. Add the mustard and sugar. Replace the lid and shake well. Store at room temperature (not in the fridge!) for up to 1 week.

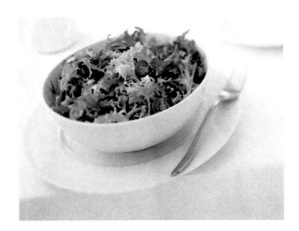

Avocado, Crab & Coriander Salad

Serves 4

Ingredients:

275g/ 10 oz frozen crab meat or canned meat
1 butter head lettuce
175g of lamb's lettuce or young spinach
1 large ripe avocado, peeled and sliced
175g/ 6oz cherry tomatoes
Black pepper and nutmeg
For the dressing
75ml/ 5tbsp extra virgin olive oil
15ml/ 1 tbsp lime juice
45ml/ 3tbsp chopped fresh coriander (optional)
½ tsp caster sugar

Method

Combine the dressing ingredients in a screw-top-jar and shake well to combine. Wash and spin the lettuces, then toss them in the dressing. Distribute the salad leaves among four plates. Top with avocado, crab meat, tomatoes. Season with pepper and nutmeg and serve.

Salad Nicoise

Serves 4

Ingredients

225g/ 8oz green beans, topped and tailed
3 eggs, hard-boiled
1 cos lettuce
120ml/ 4fl oz of French dressing – or according to taste
225g/ 8oz of plum tomatoes cut into quarters
400g/ 14oz canned tuna steak in brine
50g canned sweetcorn drained
30ml/ 2 tbsp capers - 12 black olives (optional)

Method

Boil the green beans for 6 minutes. Drain and cool the beans under running water. Wash the lettuce and spin dry then chop the leaves roughly. Moisten with half of the dressing in a large bowl. Moisten the green beans and tomatoes, sweet corn with dressing, and then scatter over the salad leaves. Break up the tuna fish with a fork and distribute over the salad with olives and capers.

Mixed bean salad

Ingredients

1 can of mixed bean
2 tomatoes chopped
50g canned sweet corn drained
3 spring onions (scallions) trimmed and chopped
125g feta cheese or 3 hard boiled eggs or 4 chicken sausages

Ingredients for dressing

3 tbsp of extra virgin olive oil
1 tbsp of mustard
1 tbsp of cumin
1 tbsp of tomato puree
Pepper

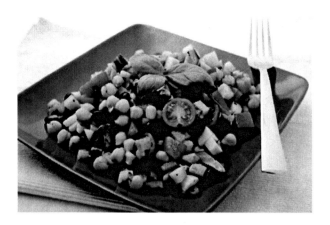

Method

Drain and wash the beans and pour into a bowl. Add the dressing to the beans. Add the sweet corn, tomatoes and spring onions and feta/boiled eggs or sausages to the bean mixture, tossing gently to coat in the dressing. Season with pepper

Harlequin chicken

Ingredients

10 skinless boneless chicken thighs
1 medium onion
1 each medium red, green and yellow (bell) peppers
1 tbsp of extra virgin olive oil
400g of can chopped tomatoes
2 tbsp chopped fresh parsley
Salad to serve

Method

Using a sharp knife cut the chicken thighs into small bite-sized pieces. Peel and thinly slice the onion. Halve and deseed the (bell) peppers and cut into small diamond shapes. Heat the oil in a shallow pan then quickly fry the chicken and onion until golden. Add the peppers, cook for 2-3 minutes, then stir in the tomatoes and chopped fresh parsley and season with pepper. Cover tightly and simmer for about 15minutes until the chicken and vegetables are tender. Serve hot with a green salad.

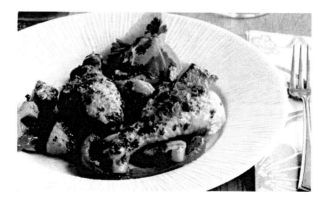

Tomato chicken with ginger

<u>Ingredients</u>

1 tbsp of extra virgin olive oil
4 chicken breast fillets cubed
100g/ 4oz cherry or small plum tomatoes, halved
1cm fresh root ginger, peeled and sliced into fine strips
1 bunch spring onions, trimmed and sliced
1-2 tsp tomato puree
Salad to serve

<u>Method</u>

Heat the oil and then cook the chicken for 5 minutes until lightly browned. Remove and set aside. Add tomatoes, ginger and spring onions to the pan and cook the tomatoes for 1-2 minutes. Return the chicken to the pan with 2 tbsp of water. Cook for 2-3 minutes until chicken is cooked through. Serve with salad.

Marinated Chicken

When in a rush, it is always great to have this in your freezer. When buying chicken breast fillets ask to have them cut into small cubes. Once home, divide them and put one half in a freezer bag with a crushed garlic glove, a bit of olive oil, juice of half a lemon and herbs de Provence. Put in the freezer and voila. With the other half you can add olive oil, cumin and pepper for a spicier chicken marinate. Again put in the freezer till you need it.

Homemade burgers:

Serves 4

<u>Ingredients</u>

500g/ 1lb2oz extra lean minced beef
1 small onion, very finely chopped
1 clove garlic, crushed
1 scant tsp dried oregano
1 tbsp wholegrain mustard
Black pepper

1 egg beaten
Serve on a bed of lettuce, with spring onions and tomatoes

Method

Put all the ingredients for the burgers (except beaten egg) into a bowl and mix well together. Add enough beaten egg to bind the ingredients together. Divide the mixture into four and shape into burgers, max 2cm in depth. Big fat burgers are tempting but it take ages to cook them right through to the middle.

To cook, heat a little hot oil on a pan and fry the burgers allowing for 6-8 minutes per side. For a cheese burger, at the end of the cooking add a slice of low fat cheese on top of the burger and let it melt nicely.

Pork stir-fry

Serve 4

Ingredients

450g lean pork, cut into thin strips
2 tbsp of light soy sauce
1-2 tbsp of olive oil
2 gloves garlic, chopped
225g of chopped vegetables (carrot in match stick size, spring onions, broccoli, cauliflowers, peas, mange-tout, baby corn, red pepper, etc…choice is endless)
50g cashew nuts (unsalted ones)

Method

Mix the pork with the soy sauce. Heat a wok or deep frying pan, add the oil, then add the garlic and pork and stir fry for 5-6 minutes. Add the vegetables. Lightly grill the cashew nuts and add on top of the vegetables. Ready to eat!

For something with a bit more flavour you can add 1 or 2 tsp of Chinese 5 spice to the vegetables add a little bit of water and stir.

Appendix 2

Stretching Plan

1.   Warm Up:

Before you begin any stretching, it's important to first warm up the muscles. Five to ten minutes of moderate physical activity will prepare your body for work and help reduce the likelihood of muscle strain. Jog lightly on the spot, use a stationary bike, jump up and down lightly, anything that gets your heart pumping and makes you start to feel hot will do.

Ideally, all exercise sessions should be followed by a few minutes of stretching. If you are stretching after exercise then you can skip the warm up above as you will probably be warm anyway!

2.   Chest and Shoulder Stretch:

Stand with your feet shoulder-width apart. Clasp hands behind your back. Straighten and raise your arms, making sure your chest doesn't collapse. Lift your chest to your chin. Hold for 15 seconds then relax. Repeat three times. You should feel a stretch in the chest and front of the shoulders.

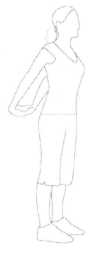

178

3.   Tall stretch

While standing or sitting, grasp
your hands together above your
head with your palms up and
shoulders relaxed. Stretch arms
up. Don't hold your breath or arch
your back. Hold for 15 seconds.
This is a good stretch to do
anytime, anywhere. You should
feel a stretch in your arms and
upper back.

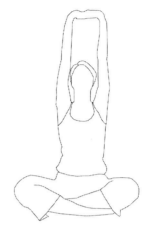

4.   Calf Stretch

Stand with one foot in front of the
other. Bend the front leg while
keeping the back leg straight and
push your back heel to the floor.
Bend your forward knee until a
comfortable stretch is felt in your
back calf. You can hold on to a wall
or chair for balance. Hold for 15
seconds.

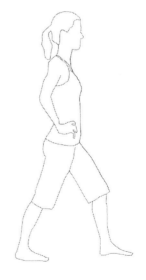

5. Seated Hamstring Stretch

Sit with one leg straight out in front, and the other leg bent with the foot against the inner thigh. Leaning forward from the hips, reach hands down the leg as far as comfortable, keeping the back as straight as possible. Do not round the back while leaning forward. Reach toward the toes. Hold the stretch for 15 seconds. Repeat two to three times for each leg. You should feel this stretch in your lower back and/or at the backs of your thighs (hamstrings)

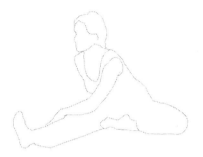

6. Standing Lower Back Stretch

Stand with your feet hip-width apart, feet firmly planted on the ground, with your hands supporting your lower back and keeping your chin to your chest. Gently arch your back. Hold for 15 seconds. You should feel a stretch in your lower back and possibly the front hips.

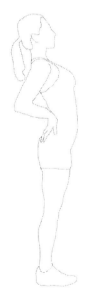

7.   *Quadriceps stretch*

Balance or use a stable object for support. Stand straight and grasp your right foot with your left hand behind you. Gently pull your foot towards your buttocks until you feel a gentle stretch down the front of your leg. Hold for 15 seconds then relax. Repeat three times on each leg. If you can't reach your foot, you can hold on to your pants or socks.

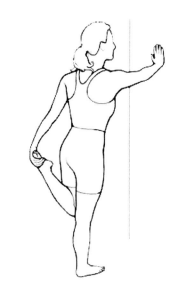

8.   *Tuck Stretch*

Lie on the floor or on a bed. Pull your knees to your chest. Push your lower back towards the ground and hold for 15 seconds. Relax and repeat three times.

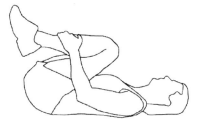

9.   *Lower Back Rotation Stretch*

Sit as shown in diagram: left leg straight, right leg crossing over left leg with right foot on the floor. Place your left elbow on the outside of bent right leg and right hand behind you. Turn your head to look over right shoulder. Hold for 15 seconds. Reverse position and look the other way. Repeat twice on each side.

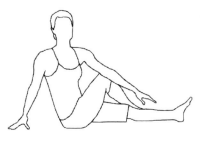

10. Back and Shoulder Stretch

Hold your left wrist with your right hand behind your back. Lean your right ear to your right shoulder. The right hand pulls the left arm down and across behind your back. You should feel a stretch in your left-side neck and shoulder. Hold stretch for 15 seconds then relax. Repeat three times on each side.

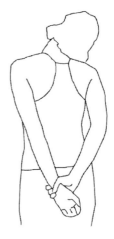

11. Quadriceps and Groin Stretch

Kneel on the floor, step forward until the front knee is over your ankle and the other knee is resting on the floor. Lower front hip downwards without moving knee position. You should feel an easy stretch in the front hip and thigh of the back leg. Hold for 15 seconds. Repeat three times for each leg. Hold on to a chair for balance if needed.

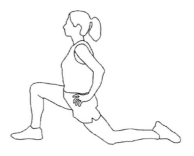

12. Word of Caution

If you have had a previous injury, are currently injured or are unsure of how to undertake these stretches safely, please check these stretches with your doctor, other qualified health professional or specialist. Do not stretch to the point of pain. Stretches should be gentle and slow, never bouncy or fast.

Appendix 3

Additional Resistance Training Exercises

1. Exercises for the Chest

Flat Dumbbell Bench Press
(works the chest muscles and triceps)

1. Lying flat on bench, hold the dumbbells directly above chest with the arms extended.
2. Lower dumbbells to chest in a controlled manner.
3. Press dumbbells back to starting position and repeat.
4. Avoid locking the elbows at the end of the movement.

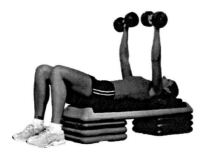

Incline Chest Presses
(concentrates work on the upper chest, shoulders and triceps)

1. Adjust the bench to an incline of between 30 to 45 degrees.
2. Repeat as explained above for the flat bench press.

Flat Chest Flies
(works the chest area independent of the triceps)

1. Lying flat on bench, hold dumbbells directly above chest.

2. Bend elbows slightly and maintain this bend throughout the exercise.
3. Open arms to sides. Elbows should remain 'locked' in a slightly bent position.
4. When the upper arms are parallel to floor, return the weights to the starting position and repeat.

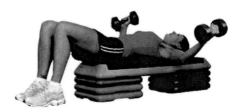

2. Exercises for the Shoulders

Seated Dumbbell Shoulder Presses
(works the entire shoulder muscles)

1. Sit upright on bench or ball with dumbbells held above your head. Make sure the back is flat.
2. Lower dumbbells slowly to shoulders.
3. When arms are at 90 degrees, press the dumbbells back up and repeat.

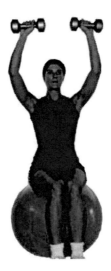

Lateral Raises
(works the top of the shoulders)

1. Stand upright, knees slightly bent, shoulder width apart, holding dumbbells at sides.
2. Bend elbows slightly and raise the dumbbells out to the sides. Keep the elbows slightly bent throughout.
3. When the arms are parallel to floor, slowly lower back and repeat.

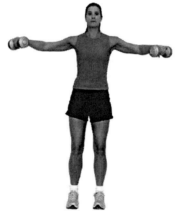

Reverse Flies
(works the back of the shoulders)

1. Sit on the edge of bench with your feet flat on the floor. Bend over so the chest is almost resting on thighs.
2. Hold the dumbbells next to your feet and bend your arms slightly. Open the arms out while keeping elbows bent.
3. When the arms are parallel to floor, slowly lower the dumbbells back.

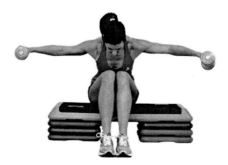

Front Raises
(works the front of the shoulders)

1. Stand upright with the knees slightly bent and feet shoulder width apart. Palms should be towards the thighs.
2. Raise one dumbbell directly in front of you.
3. When the arm is parallel to ground lower dumbbell slowly back down to the starting position. Repeat with the other arm.

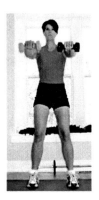

Upright Rows
(works the neck, shoulders and biceps)

1. Stand upright, feet shoulder width apart, knees slightly bent.
2. Keeping dumbbells close to body, raise them to chin.
3. Hold for a count of 2 and slowly lower to start position and repeat.

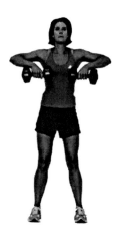

3.   <u>Exercises for the Upper Back</u>

Single Arm Row
(works the upper back)

1. Stand upright next to a bench. Place one knee and hand on bench. The Upper body should be parallel to floor.
2. Hold one dumbbell with arm extended.
3. Raise dumbbell up to your midsection keeping back still throughout movement.
4. Slowly lower dumbbell to start position and repeat.

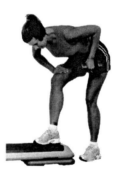

Alternating Dumbbell Bent-over Rows
(works the upper back)

1. Bend over at the waist until your torso is parallel to floor or at 45 degree angle, pull your stomach in and make sure your knees are slightly bent.
2. Hold the dumbbells straight down without locking the elbows.
3. Bend the right elbow and pull the arm up until it is level with the torso.
4. Lower the arm and immediately repeat the exercise with the left arm, keeping the movements slow and controlled.

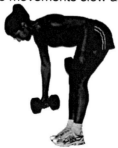

4.   Exercises for the Lower Back

Straight Leg Dead Lifts
(works the lower back, buttocks and legs)
1. Stand upright, feet shoulder width apart, knees slightly bent and hold dumbbells in front of your thighs.
2. Keeping the shoulders back, stomach pulled in and the back straight, bend from the hips and lower the weights towards the floor.
3. Lower as far as your flexibility allows. Keep looking forward throughout the exercise.
4. Stand upright using lower back and legs, maintaining a flat back and keeping your head up.

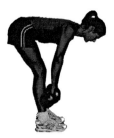

Dumbbell Squats
(works the buttocks and legs)
1. Holding dumbbells (with palms inward), stand with feet hip-width apart; don't lock knees.
2. Keeping your weight on your heels, contract your abdominal muscles and bend your knees, lowering your upper torso. Don't go lower than the illustration shows.
3. Slowly straighten up; repeat.

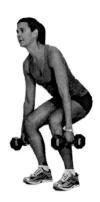

5.   Exercises for the Arms

Incline Seated Bicep Curls
(works the biceps - front of the upper arms)

1. Sit on a bench that has been adjusted to a 45 degree incline or use an exercise ball.
2. Hold dumbbells at sides. Arms should be fully extended.
3. Keep elbows close to body and curl weight up by bending the elbows

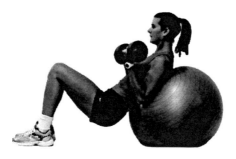

Preacher Curls
(works the biceps – front of the upper arms)

1. Set bench so back rest is approx 45 degrees or use an exercise ball.
2. Stand behind the bench. Holding the dumbbell, rest the back of upper arm on back rest or ball, with the arm fully extended.
3. Keep the back of the upper arm against the back rest or ball and curl the dumbbell up towards your face.

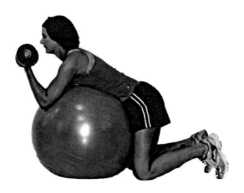

Seated Triceps Extensions
(works the triceps – back of the upper arms)
1. Sit on a bench or ball and hold a medium weight at one end with both hands overlapping one another.
2. Take the weight straight up overhead with the arms kept next to the ears.
3. Lower the weight behind the head until elbows are at about a 90 degree angle.
4. Squeeze the triceps to straighten the arms without locking the joints.

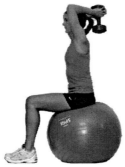

Triceps Kickbacks
(works the triceps – back of the upper arms)
1. Hold a dumbbell in each hand and bend over until your torso is at a 45-degree angle or parallel to the floor. Bend the knees if needed and keep the stomach pulled in to protect the lower back.
2. Begin the movement by bending the arms and pulling the elbows up to torso level.
3. Holding that position, straighten the arms out behind you, squeezing the triceps muscles.
4. Bend the arms back to starting position and repeat.

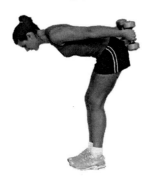

Lightning Source UK Ltd.
Milton Keynes UK
UKOW052148191011

180604UK00003B/2/P